T0149989

healed

A divinely inspired path
to overcoming cancer

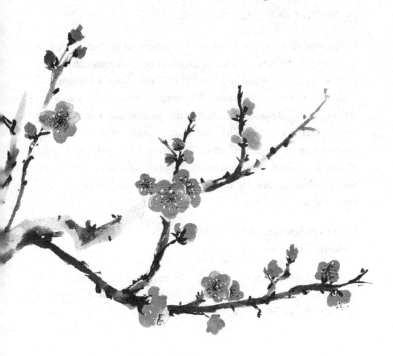

Pamela Herzer, M.A.

healed

A Divinely Inspired Path to Overcoming Cancer

Difference Press, Washington, D.C., USA
© Pamela Herzer, 2019

ISBN: 978-1-68309-266-7

Cover Design: Jennifer Hoffman Essen
Editing: Cory Hott

Scripture quotation taken from the Authorized King James Version. Quotations taken from *Science and Health with Key to the Scriptures* by Mary Baker Eddy.

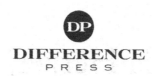

DIFFERENCE PRESS

I dedicate this book to my children,

Colleen and John.

Thank you for giving me the will to live.

I love you with all my heart.

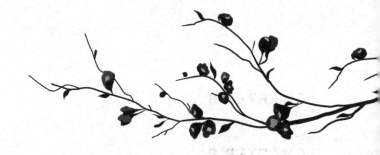

Table Of Contents

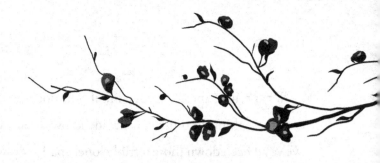

Foreword

Let me ask you a few questions.

What will it be like for you to feel thoroughly loved to your bones, because of divine Love?

What will it mean for you to connect intimately with God in your next crisis when you feel helpless and all alone? And the outcome would be successful and complete healing?

What would it be like to hear someone assuring you that you are deserving of all love every moment and this would wipe away all of your self-doubts and fears?

What would it mean to receive 100 percent support for your emotional, physical, and spiritual well-being, to be seen as a masterpiece?

How would it feel to go from devastation to total confidence while, along the way, becoming the person of light who you truly are?

Oh, one more question.

What will it mean in your life if you don't experience these things? I think you already know the answer. We've all been down those terribly lonely paths, drowning in our hopelessness and bewildered by our scary condition, wondering about the possibilities of hope and healing while coming up empty handed.

I don't wish to scare you with the last question, but I do want you to consider your bigger life possibilities through the porthole of a qualified healer who has walked the walk and is devoted to healing – and a proven spiritual warrior – through her alignment with Love. In these pages, you will discover the glorious life that waits for you to discover it. A life beyond the usual victim status and a life of becoming a spiritual warrior yourself. Didn't ask for that? What if I told you that this is the requirement for being healed of a fatal disease, and that it was possible?

Congratulations on investing in yourself by picking up *Healed: A Divinely Inspired Path to Overcoming Cancer* by Pamela Herzer, M.A. It's a rare account of a woman who considers herself to be "a messenger of light and love," and clearly proves it, page after page. You'll feel the love; it gives hope to us all.

Each chapter is a deeper step into your glorious self, led by a woman who is able to show you how to step outside of the worst possible diagnoses of cancer, which included healing herself from the toxicity of a marriage, her dad ignoring her for many years, a violent assault of attempted rape, self-hate, and more. Pam has experienced the worst of the worst. Not only did she find the key to healing through the power of divine Love, but she also learned to use her most deplorable relationships, deep wounds, and lack of self-esteem as a springboard for higher learning and her soul's ascension.

Through her personal story, written intimately and passionately for the reader, she succeeds in lighting up the reader with a promise of a world of hope, healing, and a new life created from taking the divine path.

As I read through the book, I found myself reignited with my deep love for God, my primal passion to serve, and to remember why I am here, and to recommit to the finest and best life I know by staying close to divine Love.

You deserve a rich and wonderful life, full of love and healing. Pam will take you by the hand and show you how to move out of great darkness into radiant light, just as she herself did. Her steps are simple, profound, and proven.

It's time for you to be divinely inspired to overcome your worst fears – including a medical diagnosis of cancer (or any disease) – and to be healed.

Sending you all love!

SHANNON PECK

Author of *Love Heals: How to Heal Everything with Love*, co-author of *The Love You Deserve: A Spiritual Guide to Genuine Love*, and co-founder of TheLoveCenter.com

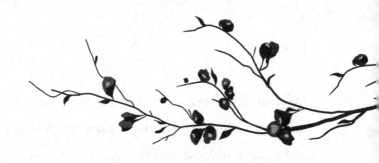

Introduction

Y ou're going about your life, then you get a call from your doctor that changes your life forever. Your mood shifts. Fear takes over your body, and you look like a deer caught in headlights. All of a sudden, your life passes in front of your face, and you know that the cancer diagnosis you just received is a gamechanger. You feel that life as you know it is gone forever.

This happened to me, and I went into a dark, black hole of depression. Where do I begin, and who do I talk to? Do I call my parents? Should we call a family meeting? Maybe I should call my best friend. Perhaps my minister should know. What doctors or healers should I contact? What these questions are really referring to is, "who can I talk to to take this whole nightmare away? Someone, please tell me this just isn't true, because I can't handle this fear and pressure."

Through this book, you will feel incredibly empowered to go through this experience with a deep knowing that the diagnosis is here for your growth and ascension. You will meet angels along the way to help and guide you. Most importantly, you will get to know yourself as God knows you, made in the image and likeness of impeccable Love.

We will address how gratitude and forgiveness are vital to healing. You will be reassured that you have power and dominion over your thoughts. In fact, you'll learn to have the thoughts of God when you align with Him. What would it feel like to know you are not a victim of your circumstances? I felt powerful when I learned how to give gratitude to God for my life lesson, cancer, because I got to grow closer to divine Love and do the work that I signed up to do before I arrived on this Earth plane. God doesn't bring us cancer but, She certainly delivers us from cancer.

I am not here to heal you, but instead, to lead you to the heart of Love where all healing resides; in your heart. I am simply a messenger. I make no promises to heal anyone or anything. I had to do this for myself and wouldn't have missed it for the world. I am now here for you as your guidance counselor, if you will, to lead you out of the pit of despair and to the arms of Love.

I use the words God, Spirit, Love, divine Love, and Source interchangeably to mean the same thing. God is both masculine and feminine, hence, the usage of Him, Her, His, She, Mother, and Father.

This is my gift of love for humanity. It is my time to pay forward what I learned in the hopes that you too can learn to align with divine Love and move through the ever-fearful waters of cancer.

It is with a servant's heart that I offer the story of my divinely inspired path to healing my own cancer. May you be in health and prosper!

chapter 1

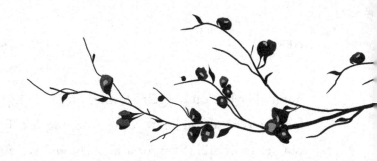

Life Can Change in
the Blink of an Eye

L et's face it, the word *cancer* is a scary one. It can send you into a tailspin and paralyze your thinking. The word tests you in ways sometimes beyond what we think we can handle. We come face-to-face with our mortality and do a reassessment of our whole life. Sometimes we go into an emotional rage, sometimes we shut down. Some become energized and warrior-like. One wants to fight it out and slay the dragon named cancer. Others want to stay in bed and never get out because of the feelings and emotions cancer brings up for them. Remembering people who have struggled with a cancer diagnosis makes them feel hopeless.

You've just received the news you have cancer. It's a scary time, and your heart is racing. I understand. It's okay to become emotional. It's possible that you feel numb. Maybe I can suggest a loving, self-honoring way for you to be so you know you're not alone. See if you can get really still. Stop for a moment and get quiet. It's okay, do this when you're ready. Tenderly listen to Love. A thought comes to you that says it is time to let go of old, outdated ways of thinking, and time for the new healing thoughts to flood your consciousness. After all, to feel the total peace that comes with divine Love is what our hearts call out for above anything else.

Allow yourself to bathe in the warm, silky waters of Love, and experience the infinite possibilities of a new life, one of health and joyful living. Ponder for a moment that cancer is an opportunity for true growth and a stepping stone to a higher, more aligned way of living. It is one that will set you on a new path of a deeper love for yourself. It will cause you to be of fuller service to humanity and, most importantly, a radical commitment to God's abundant will for your life. Let's roll up our sleeves and get to work. You are worth the effort. Let's again remember, a cancer diagnosis is an opportunity for true growth, not a life sentence.

Let's take a moment and examine your thinking. What is in your consciousness? This is the most important step. You might think that you should first run to a doctor, tell your partner, sit down with your children, or have a heart-to-heart conversation with your best friend or sister, but there is definitely a "first step" to take that would be more efficient and save a lot of time. Dropping from your head to your heart should be your first go-to. Understanding that all the well-meaning people in your life cannot take away the pain and scariness that the word cancer brings up. So, we go to our heart-of-love, where all answers reside and where divine Love is, waiting for the invitation from you to begin a life. Waiting for you to step fully and consciously into a life aligned with the way God sees and knows you. Spirit has been graciously waiting for you to understand that the kingdom of heaven is within you. Love has been patiently waiting and now receives you with open arms. We love the people in our lives, but they can never do for us what divine Love does. You don't get to heaven in twos. You get to heaven only with your hand in God's, in alignment with Him/Her. This is your life. We can't afford to water it down with opinions and fears of others.

What causes you not to feel God's love? Does this all sound like a pie-in-the-sky approach to healing cancer? Were you raised in a religion that limited your thinking and is based in fear and damnation? Perhaps you weren't raised in any particular religion at all, and you feel like a boat without a rudder. Maybe you reject the word "religion" and prefer spirituality. Many people I work with have studied and appreciated a more enlightened sense of the Bible and their relationship to Spirit. They prefer knowing God as Love and not as an anthropomorphic God who sits in the clouds judging everyone. The same people know a spiritual foundation and a spiritual law governs their lives and they cast their net fully in that direction.

Do you think you can suspend, for a moment, the lens you looked through on this journey called life and your cancer diagnosis? Can you simply ponder what it means to be the most cherished daughter or son of the Most High? Would you be willing to pause for a moment and not judge cancer as good or bad? Simply observe the diagnosis and not absorb it. This action will put you in a more quiet place of dominion over the problem and not in the middle of it. Do you realize that you have the chance to make your relationship with God the way you want it instead of the thought or religion you were raised in? Would you like to begin anew? I bet you're ready to know Love in a fuller, more expansive way now. Can you trust your gut regarding

God? "Putting on the new man" takes exactly that; changing your thought to align with what God knows about you, "made in the image and likeness" of God, divine Love.

Are you in a difficult marriage? Do you look for your partner to show empathy for your tender heart, especially after being told you have cancer? Is he too busy with work and golf to sit with you while you process your pain? Does he keep an emotional distance from you for whatever reason? Do you just need someone to take away all the emotional and physical pain you experience, even for a moment? Do you feel lonely in your marriage, like the well of your heart is dried up and there is no more joy, lightness, and levity? Perhaps you feel resentful of your partner for not delivering on all the promises he made at one time.

Maybe you're mad at yourself for getting into such a relationship and you feel stuck. "Should I stay or should I go?" seems to be your daily mantra. When he walks into the room, your teeth clench, your throat constricts, and you feel that pit in your stomach. The way we relate to the people and circumstances of our lives determine our health and happiness. I understand because the marriage I describe was my marriage.

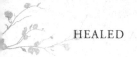

I felt lonely, misunderstood, but most of all, lost. I wanted my husband to tenderly hold me and comfort me after I was diagnosed with cancer. I thought he intentionally withheld his love from me and alienated me. Come to find out, he simply didn't know how to do the things I needed him to do. I now see that the resentment I felt for my husband contributed to me getting sick. Holding a grudge for too long is not healthy. My body manifested the loathing and hatred I felt for my husband. Hatred equals cancer. It was time for me to change my relationship to the way I experienced my husband's behavior.

Do you expect your children to be perfect human beings? Do you expect them to excel at everything they do regarding their grades in school, sports teams, and popularity? Do you stress while working to get them into the best schools? Does your heart sink when you see your child suffer? In other words, do you empathize with your child to the degree that you carry the weight of your child's pain? This can feel like there is no separation between you and your child.

I suffered tremendously because of this. I felt my daughter's struggle with her friendships. I also felt the sadness my son felt when his dad and I finally separated. Women think they need to go on a diet to lose excess pounds when it is the excessive fear and stress they carry. Spiritually speaking, excess weight equals excess fear, heaviness of thought and the weightiness of the world. Parents think they are responsible for everything that happens to their child. This causes them to beam when their child "succeeds" and fall apart when their child "fails." What would it feel like to see them through divine Love's eyes, knowing you are your children's earthly guardian, but God is their true parent? Never do we shirk our duties as their earthly parent but, instead, we align with divine Love as our true parent to know how to parent better.

What is the desire of your heart at this moment? Tap into your massive heart of love and listen. Tender, Christly compassion for yourself is crucial. Relating to yourself independent of all judgment is paramount to your healing. Can you allow yourself to feel like God's masterpiece? You have the choice to think the opposite, but I don't recommend you do that. You are too precious. You are one of a kind. God needs you. Everyone asks, "What is my purpose?" Your purpose is simply to glorify God in everything you do. This isn't old theology. It is current, relevant thinking. When

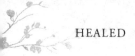

one glorifies God in everything you do, we then know what our purpose is.

Dear friend, believe me, I know what you're going through. I have been diagnosed with cancer. I have walked the walk. I tried traditional and nontraditional healing methods and got more sick and tired until I found the exact answer I needed to live. Many nights I cried myself to sleep, only to wake the next day in a zombie-like stupor. I exhausted myself carrying the weight of fear.

I stand shoulder to shoulder with you, dear friend. Many years later, I live an abundantly happy and healthy life. I healed my cancer by a method I have affectionately named Aligning With the Divine. It has proven to be the most immediate and effective method I've ever experienced.

Know that I see you. I care deeply and feel your cry for help. I've walked in your shoes in that dark and dusty valley. I came out the other end whole and aligned. This same healing is here for you, too.

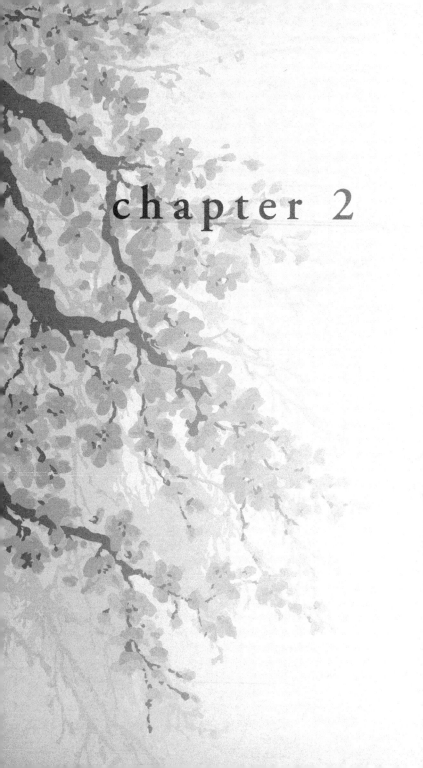

chapter 2

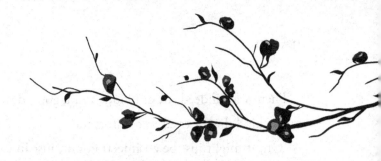

I Understand.
I've Been There.

THE DAY MY LIFE
CHANGED FOREVER

I was scared out of my mind and paralyzed with fear when I noticed the fresh blood after intercourse, which was odd because I had just finished my period. These things don't happen to me. I'm a good person. I don't have a mean bone in my body. Why me, and why now?

I made an appointment with a gynecologist. As I lay on the cold, crunchy table from the white sterile paper that covered the table I said, "This stuff happens to other people, not me. I'm healthy. Other people get cancer. I don't." All of this went through my mind before the doctor said anything to me. It was completely surreal.

There was, indeed, fresh blood, and a good deal of it. The kind doctor tried to comfort me.

"Oh, it might just be an infection but, just in case, we should get a biopsy."

The day came to get that biopsy and it hurt. I cried. I was lonely. My whole life crumbled before my eyes. I fell into a deep pit of despair and I just wanted the nightmare to go away. Here I was, at the same age, diagnosed with the same cancer as Carla, my first husband's late wife – a seasoned spiritual thinker who belonged to a church that emphasized healing by prayer.

The biopsy showed that the cancer was present on my cervix, but the doctor didn't know how far it had spread, so he scheduled out-patient surgery to explore the situation. He did a procedure where they surgically removed the lining of my uterus a couple of inches. In the days following, the results revealed that the cancer spread into my uterus. I fell deeper into despair, and darkness covered me like a heavy raincloud. I couldn't see my way past this. The cloud was the darkest of the dark. It was wet and soggy. All my lightness simply left.

In and out of doctor's appointments left me feeling vulnerable and unsure of myself. My confidence left. I felt flawed, useless, unworthy of love and an immense distrust that there was a God.

Where was God in all of this? Why was I being punished? What an awful trick to play on me. I had two beautiful children to raise. I had things to do, places to go, and people to meet.

It was at this same time that we lost our family home in Montecito and moved into a rental property. We had no health insurance, so I nearly collapsed when the medical bills around $500,000 trickled in. One evening, my husband nonchalantly mentioned we were down to our last $5,000. This was tough to hear because the rent was due. It was $3,400 a month, which left us little to live on. I had no idea what we were going to do. Fear consumed me. My husband was emotionally absent. Perhaps he hadn't healed his grief over Carla dying. He never talked about it. This must have been hard for him to go through this again. I told him the bare minimum just to protect him, but the fact was that I hurt, and I needed comfort. We retreated to our corners because neither one of us knew how to be with this situation. I kept all my emotions inside. I used to yearn for his love and understanding, but it never came.

MORE BAD NEWS

Five days into being in the hospital, the main doctor and his assistant came into my room to give me the results from the tests they took during surgery. The doctor could barely look me in the eye when he said, "The cancer has spread. We took a number of lymph nodes from your abdomen and tested them for cancer, and they were all infected, we're sorry to say." This devastated me. My mother drove me home after being in the hospital for a week. I told my children I had a "tummy ache." They learned how to be gentle with me and let me take naps when I needed to rest.

My life, as I knew it, would have to change. I was getting ready to learn that I was "enough." I didn't have to be a people-pleaser. I didn't have to acquiesce to others to make them feel comfortable at the expense of my own happiness and for the sake of harmony. Conflict was difficult for me, so I did everything to deflect harsh emotions. I learned how to control others' experience of me just to feel safe.

MY ANGELS IN THE GLOOM

I thought the fear I felt would kill me before cancer. I emotionally fell apart with every ache and pain, thinking that the cancer had spread. I had six weeks of radiation after my hysterectomy. Again, because my husband was emotionally absent, I drove myself to the cancer clinic, put on the light grey dressing gown and joined my two technicians, Rachel and David, in the treatment room. As daunting and ominous as all the medical machines were, the two technician friends I made were my angels, encouraging me every step of the way. The machines were big and scary, but their presence kept me grounded.

Rachel and David were just two of the healing angels I needed so badly at that time. They'd greet me with, "Hey Pam, great to see you. Let's get this party started." For six weeks, they ushered me onto a steel table where they would step outside the room to maneuver the radiation machine and direct it to the little dot tattoos that were permanently inked onto my body. My abdomen looked like a landing strip for a DC-10 airplane. A little humor goes a long way in situations like this. I played a game with myself and pretended that the big machine that hovered over me was Spirit, beaming Her deep healing light inside of me to heal the cancer. My mantra became, "thank you God for healing me, thank you, God, I love you."

At the end of the six weeks of radiation, the technician, Rachel, gave me a book titled, *When I Am Old,*

I Shall Wear Purple. I wept when she handed me this most precious of books because it was Rachel's way of saying, "Hang in there. You've got this." I interpreted Rachel's gift as a wink from God saying I had a long life ahead of me and to be myself. I tightly hugged Rachel and David the last time I visited the cancer ward for my radiation treatment. I wished they could promise me that I would live but, of course, they couldn't guarantee any such thing. Instead, they gave me the book and hugged me. I believe they had been just as touched by our mutual experience as I was.

Gentle tears and warm hugs were generous that day. I will never forget my angels in the cancer treatment center in Santa Barbara, California. I drove home, walked upstairs to my husband's office looking for any kind of validation that I just completed six weeks of radiation. I experienced deep burns in my digestive system from the radiation causing much distress, but he didn't seem to notice me. He kept his head on the computer screen and grunted a little acknowledgment. I went to the bedroom and fell asleep. Was it because my body hurt or perhaps the loneliness I felt in my marriage? I didn't know. What I did know is that I needed to escape for a bit and not think or feel. I was numb.

About a month after the radiation, my doctor's staff kept calling me to get back to the cancer treatment center to start chemotherapy. By this time, after the surgeries and subsequent treatment, I couldn't do it anymore. In addition to working with my doctors, I called many people for healing. These were all well-meaning people who listed themselves as practitioners or healers. I have never known such a loving and dedicated group of people, but I just seemed to be getting worse instead of better. My heart sank when the hospital called repeatedly, urging me to start chemotherapy, but I just couldn't do it. I couldn't handle the painful procedures and the uncertainty of whether I would live or not. I was suffering and I needed to find a way, to relate to this whole cancer ordeal in a different way. I was sick and tired of being sick and tired.

A HEART BEGINNING TO OPEN

During this next phase, I began opening up to divine Love (God). From the beginning, I was so fearful that I just wanted to get this whole thing healed and get on with my life. I always loved God and felt Her presence, so why wasn't I trusting in Her care now?

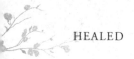

Simply put, because I was afraid, and I panicked. I had children to raise, and I was way too young to be faced with my mortality. I didn't want my mother and father to have to witness their daughter passing on. I didn't want to cause grief to those I loved. I asked God, continually, what I needed to know. Many times during the quiet of the night, the words from the Psalmist in the Bible came to my thoughts, "I shall not die, but live, and declare the works of the Lord." I clung to those words as divine Love speaking directly to me. I embraced the feeling of those words as the truth coming to me from Love's mouth. It felt like a warm stream of water washing my soul of any doubt I had. The feeling was short-lived but, in the moment, I felt the presence of God comforting and reassuring me that She needed me to live.

NINE MONTHS AFTER RADIATION

About nine months after the cancer surgery and radiation, my two children and I planned a play date with one of my best friends, Carol, and her two children. I felt strong enough that day to go out and have a little fun with my children. Colleen and John were chomping at the bit for a play date with Robby and DeeDee.

I went downstairs to pack up, and as I turned quickly, I felt something snap in my abdomen. I thought nothing of it and continued to get my kids in the car. All of a sudden I experienced an overwhelming urge to run to the bathroom and throw up. I was dizzy, lightheaded, and thought I might have either food poisoning, or a bout of the flu that came on quickly.

I immediately called Carol to cancel our playdate but instead, Carol came over to pick up my children and take them to her home. I went straight to bed, violently throwing up until there was nothing left. Anytime I tried to eat anything it came right back up, water included. I was in this condition almost a week before I realized I might be passing on. I thought I just had the flu because of the high temperature and vomiting, but come to find out it was much more dangerous than the flu.

On the sixth night, I passed in and out of consciousness. One of our dear friends, Bill, came over to the house and carried me downstairs and into the car. I remember little of this because I was groggy, at best. He rushed me to the emergency room where I waited in a wheelchair, wearing my Lanz nightgown and UGGs, holding onto my small plastic trash can just in case there might be any little amount that needed to come up. I was so weak that I couldn't hold my head up. I had been dry-heaving for days. Finally, they wheeled me into an examination room and pumped liquids into me, intravenously.

Little by little the lightheadedness, abated and I returned to consciousness. Come to find out, I didn't have the flu at all. I had contracted the virus Staphylococcus, somewhere along the way. It had settled in my abdomen where the radiation was directed. I had twisted my body six days before while preparing for the playdate, and the infection broke open and traveled through my bloodstream, infecting my whole body. I was so dehydrated that my heart began to stop; that coupled with an ongoing fever of 104 was killing me.

DIVINE LOVE ALIGNMENT

Why do I write about this? Simply put, it was an opportunity to move into alignment with divine Love and feel God's healing power and presence again. It was just another big bump in the road, but I learned a lot about resilience, determination, and grit by this time.

I learned to look the so-called devil (fear) right in the eyes and say, "I know who you are and you don't scare me," then step hard on that serpent's neck. I learned how to thank God for absolutely everything by that time even in the middle of a hellish experience. I began to pour blessings on the technicians, medical assistants, nurses, and doctors, quietly and sometimes verbally. I blessed the hospital. I blessed my bed. What did this do for me? It made me soar in thought to be immensely grateful for the staph infection, and for our good friend, Bill, who carried me to the car and into the emergency room.

Why could I possibly be grateful for yet another round of hospital visits? Because it brought me closer to God. It was a gift to be able to learn more about my relationship to divine Love, made in Her image and likeness. It was an honor to glorify Her even in the midst of another life-threatening experience. Gratitude is the greatest healer and when we feel love for God, our body naturally feels this. In my case, I healed quickly because of that.

After five days in the hospital, they released me with all kinds of paraphernalia attached to the area where the infection was. I wore loose clothing, rested a lot, and became more energized a little more every day. Giving gratitude became natural for me, but I was still fearful.

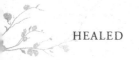

THE TURNING POINT

I was home about a week after my hospital stay when I experienced the most sacred experience. While sitting on the floor, folding laundry, I raised my head and called out to God saying, "Please help me, dear God. I am so tired of being sick and tired. Please take away this fear I'm feeling and heal me. Thank you, God. I love you, God. I know you are here with me now." My head dropped to my knees as my focus completely turned inward to my heart. Time stood still. With my eyes closed, I saw, in my mind's eye, a silhouette of Jesus Christ. I crossed the veil of matter into the realm of Spirit. Peace permeating the whole of me, washing me of every vestige of fear is the only way I can describe it. In other words, "the peace which passest all understanding."

I experienced an unadulterated and pure communion with the greatest love in the world and, all along, it was inside of me. I went from debilitating fear to the most palpable love I have ever known. I felt a soft, thin veil brush gently over my face. I don't know if this experience happened in a split second or five minutes. Again, time stood still, and I was in awe and reverence for divine Love filling all space and becoming the only power of my life. I was infinitely changed in that moment. All that existed was pure love.

I rose up from being on the floor and as I did the words flew out of my mouth, "Dear, God if I have ten more minutes to live, let me glorify You in everything I do." I felt like Moses before the burning bush. My body was electrified. I was hot to the touch. I could feel my face beaming and the smile on my face and the light in my eyes because they were fully radiant with divine Love. I had my marching orders now; if I have only ten more minutes to live, I will glorify God in everything I do. I stepped into the abyss of not knowing if I was going to live or die, but I was going to go out with a bang if I wasn't to stay on this earth. I trusted divine Love to catch me and hold me secure in Her bosom. She did just that, and there has been no turning back.

DO EVERYTHING WITH LOVE

I gently walked downstairs, still feeling shaky and weak, but I needed to wash the kitchen dishes. My body was weak, but my spiritual core was strong. I laughed when I said to myself, "Okay body, I'm going downstairs to wash the dishes, if you want to come, then let's go, but I'm going anyway." I stood at the kitchen sink feeling

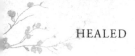

as if I was a different person, washing the dishes with immense gratitude and joy. I was fully in the present moment doing everything with love. I naturally took the most mundane task of washing dishes and meticulously infused the process with love. Tears of gratitude streamed down my face because I had the strength to wash the dishes for my family. I knew at that moment I was a new person and that life as I knew was going to be different.

When the Bible instructs me to "put on the new man after His likeness," I sit up and take notice. The opportunity to ponder what this means was life-altering. Instead of being a people-pleaser, I became a God-pleaser. I learned to drop any self-loathing and to see myself through God's eyes, made in the image and likeness of Her. What a mind-blowing concept. Think of what it means to be God's masterpiece and that every hair on your head is numbered by God. Our names are written on the palms of His hands. That's how intimate our relationship is with Love. Love is breathing in us every moment of the day. Our hearts beat in tandem with Spirit. We are one with God, so I asked myself, "if God doesn't have cancer then why do I have to have cancer?" I began to understand that I am made with the same material God is. She is spirit so I am spiritual. I also cherish the idea that God made all and pronounced it "very good." There was no "goodness" in the diagnosis called cancer.

UNSTOPPABLE

Healing ideas flowed into my consciousness. I thought, "my cup runneth over," so what shall I do with the overflow? Then I remembered the nighttime promises from God, "ye shall not die, but live and declare the works of the Lord." I learned how to talk to God like He was my best friend. I asked Love how to best serve Her and what it meant to "declare the works of the Lord." The answer didn't come at that moment, but I trusted that I would hear an answer when I needed to know how to pay forward what I learned. I took the words from I Thessalonians at face value, "pray without ceasing, and in everything, give thanks." Praying simply meant that I could talk with God like I would talk with my parent, best friend, and constant companion.

I also learned that gratitude for everything gives us the spiritual altitude to feel God's love. A beautiful verse from a beloved textbook of mine writes, "let us feel the divine energy of Spirit bringing us into new-ness of life…" (Science and Health with Key to the Scriptures by Mary Baker Eddy). I not only thought about divine Love, but I actually felt God/Spirit. This is what ultimately healed me – feeling the yumminess of God, allowing God to love me, and understanding how loved I am. This all gave me purpose. I felt buoyed and ready to live.

My body did not heal overnight. It took a number of months to regulate and normalize itself. I gained normal weight, the dizziness and lightheadedness dissi-pated, and my energy came back. I realized that it was not my energy, but instead, it was me living in align-ment with Spirit, as Her image and likeness, so I had a sufficient and lasting source of energy.

MY NEW PURPOSE

God has opened the floodgates of opportunity and filled my life with grace. I've stepped up onto a higher rung on the ascending ladder, heavenward. Now, I am doing the work I came to earth to do as Love's mes-senger, using my story of healing as support for those going through the same challenge.

I speak on stage to large and small audiences about the healing power of God and the necessity of aligning with Love for the ultimate healing. I coach amazing individuals who are ready to step into their own heart of love where all answers reside. I never give advice, because I honor and respect each person's unique relationship with God.

That said, I offer a method of aligning with divine Love that surpasses all other healing modalities that I have tried. Using my method of aligning has healed me of a sense of co-dependency with men, helped me have a lighter heart while parenting my children, and helped me to lightly hold the challenges of life rather than holding on to them so tightly. When you're aligned, you trust the answers you're getting within. You stop looking outside yourself for answers. I never discourage people from doing what they need to do to heal, but I always encourage them to check in with Love and make a decision from that vantage point.

My prayer for you is that you may know that you are enough. Your cancer story can end on a high note of healing. You can feel genuine empowerment and hopefulness on the hardest day. Yes, this will test you, but I learned how to use cancer as an opportunity instead of a death sentence, and you can too.

Again, where is God in all of this mess? Let's join hands and walk this path together.

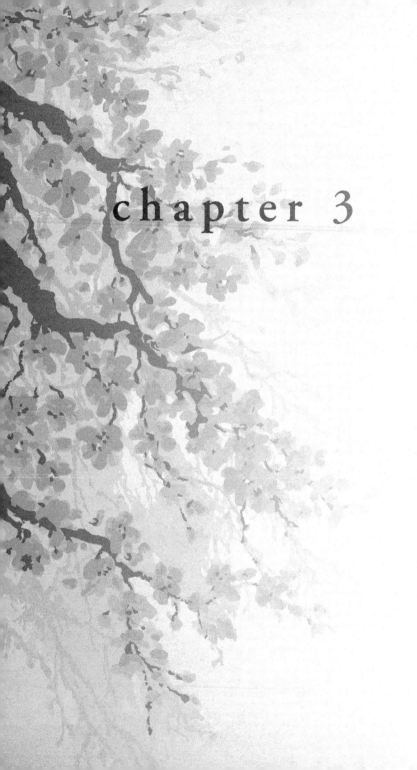

chapter 3

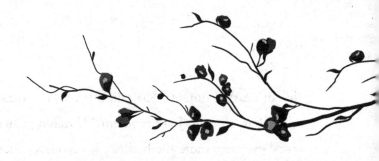

A Fresh and Inspired Approach to Healing

CHELSEA

Chelsea found me on social media. She was highly skeptical, yet receptive. She was diagnosed with breast cancer and her marriage was falling apart. Her children were giving her a fit by acting badly. I knew her children's behavior was in direct relation to the chaos in the home.

I knew I wanted to help her, but wasn't sure she would be a good fit for me. I work with clients who are ready to jump into the abyss of not knowing with both feet and trust God. Chelsea had a few not-so-good experiences with organized religion and had a chip on her shoulder. She renounced all religion and turned her back on God. She was confronted with (in her words) a "life or death moment." She said this was her "make it or break it, come to Jesus moment." Coaching Chelsea was slower and more methodical. It becomes easier to spiritually intuit my client's thoughts for the purpose of knowing the best way to work with them for the most healing results.

Chelsea chose alternative routes to heal her cancer. She used herbs, salt baths, Chinese medicine, reiki, lymphatic massage therapy, and other modalities. I told her I had zero judgment on what she chose but shared that I had tried all the same things to no avail until I learned to align with divine Love. She then chose a medical route to treat her cancer. As a coach, I stood an arm's length away, ready to help if she needed me.

One day I noticed an email request from Chelsea to schedule a chat with me. I was grateful to see this. As we talked, she cried. She was tired of being in fear. She was exhausted as she strove to keep her husband happy and her children healthy (as if it were her job). Chelsea metaphorically crumbled as she spoke like a tired child falling into the arms of an unconditionally loving parent.

"Please help me, Pam. I'm ready. I'm really, really ready now." What she needed was not me at all. She reached out to Love to comfort her aching heart and put her on the right path to wholeness and freedom. She yearned to be identified as the gorgeous and radiantly healthy child-of-God that God made instead of a flawed and sickly cancer patient.

My eyes welled up as I listened to her story. I felt enormous Christly compassion for her, but I made sure I didn't believe her story of woe. Why? Because I wouldn't have been any help to her. I have learned as a coach to be with my client or patient, but not in my client. I need to be a clear conduit for Spirit, spotless and unscathed from the world. I am a messenger of light and love. To do my work, in service to God, I must be "strong in the Lord."

It took a number of weeks before Chelsea believed that she was not the angry mother she thought she was. Anger had just become a bad habit. She realized she lost herself along the way, and I was happy to guide her back to the right path of happiness. Chelsea felt the weight of the world and the responsibility for her children's success. Her daughter was failing math and her son was falling through the cracks at school. Her husband nearly gave up on the marriage because she was never happy. I was thrilled when Chelsea decided

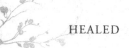

to wholeheartedly jump into the process of aligning as she trusted me by this time. I had her back, and she knew it.

Her resistance lessened as she cherished herself for the first time in her life. Her relationship with Love blossomed as we worked together to forgive herself for thinking she had to be a perfect woman. She got to the point where she stopped being codependent, looking to her husband to make every decision for the family because she didn't trust herself. Chelsea stopped blaming herself for her children's challenges and, instead, found the help she needed for them without thinking their problems were the result of something she did wrong.

Her countenance softened and her character was renewed. In the months that we worked together, she learned to delegate to her children and husband household chores that she had done with resentment for years. She learned to do "less" as she aligned with Love more. This caused her to relax and stress less. Chelsea became one of the most changed people I had ever worked with.

The moment Chelsea was ready to take the leap, Love was there with one big, loving net to catch her. I was honored to assist her in that process.

I coached her to ask herself the bigger questions: What is God? Who is she in relation to God?

Chelsea was extremely fearful that she was going to die. We needed to address the fear first and foremost. I wanted her to know that no matter how fearful she was, God was so much bigger than her problem, and she could lean on God as her ever-present help. It was a wonderful time of getting to know more about God and Her everlasting love for Chelsea. Once her fear abated, she was able to think more clearly. Aligning with divine Love comes down to one thing; what does God know about me? Then we align ourselves mentally, emotionally, physically, and spiritually with what God knows about us.

It was beautiful how Chelsea was incredibly receptive to new ways of thinking and ultimately answering those questions. I shared new ways of relating to her problems and let her know that her challenges were not present to make her life miserable, but instead, to advance in her ascension process and grow closer to divine Love. Chelsea felt breast cancer represented a damaged relationship with her children because of the pain and disfigurement of her breasts. We turned all that around by understanding that she was "made in the image and likeness" of God. I shared with her that God's mothering breasts nourish Her children and give them the perfect amount, and she could go to God as her Mother to comfort and nourish her.

It was a beautiful and fruitful time with Chelsea. Her family life turned around and her marriage is a happy one now. Last time we talked, she shared with me that her cancer is in remission and life has stabilized.

Let me break down my method of aligning with divine Love so it makes more sense and feels more rooted and grounded. What you will learn in this book is the most loving and self-honoring thing we can do for ourselves, let alone the best way to honor divine Love. My intention is to make aligning more palatable and easier to understand. I found that this method is the most reliable and practical way of dealing with any and all challenges. For the purpose of this book, where I focus on the healing of cancer, I offer how I aligned with divine Love and eventually healed myself of cancer. The following is a summation. The more one practices aligning with the divine, the easier it becomes.

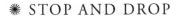

✳ STOP AND DROP

You are given a diagnosis, and your life feels like it's over. Your mind races as you think about all other people in your life who have had to go what you're going through, and fear takes over. This is the time to stop all fearful thinking and drop to your knees. The most important thing to do when fear knocks at your door is to stop it in its tracks. When you feel weak and sick to your stomach, it is time to kick fear to the curb before it finds a permanent home in your consciousness.

Remember not to give fear any oxygen. Don't give it an audience. You have total control and dominion over fear whether or not you believe this. Yes, it's scary to hear the word "cancer," but you are not a victim to it. This is your opportunity to readjust and realign your life to God as Life.

✳ MOVE INTO YOUR HEART

Immediately move into your heart of love where all answers lie. We tend to run to our friends or partners and cry on their shoulder. There is nothing wrong with this, but let's remember that they can make you feel good for a moment, but it's temporary, and the real

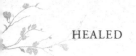

healing comes from trusting the answers you are getting from Spirit. God's voice is the only voice. God's will is the only will.

When you commune with Love, you will understand that God is the only ever-present comforter. You will feel the deepest love on this earth. When you center yourself in your heart, ask divine Love what She knows about you, how She made you. Ask Her if cancer is Her will for you. I bet you'll be pleasantly surprised at the answers you receive in the form of words, a feeling, or a simple knowing. Remember, "the kingdom of heaven is within."

✳ BREATHE

Keep breathing. We tend to hold our breath and even stop breathing when the proverbial boogie man shows up. Focus on your breath, as it will bring you into the present moment. It will keep you focused on your heart where Love resides.

You breathe the breath-of-life, so breathe deeply. After you fill your lungs with air, hold your breath for four to five seconds, then breathe out through your mouth with intention.

Breathe in with your nose, breathe out with your mouth.

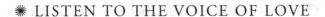

✳ LISTEN TO THE VOICE OF LOVE

You are now seated or lying down (in my case I was sitting on my knees on the floor). You now know you have the power to observe fear, but not absorb it. Your breath is a source of comfort because it's causing you to stay in the moment. Now is the time to turn to God wholeheartedly. This is your opportunity to melt into Love's arms just as a child goes to their mother to look for comfort and reassurance. Don't be shy, just do it. It's not silly. It doesn't mean you're weak. It simply means that we become as little children and turn to the strong, yet gentle arms of your divine parent.

Now allow God to speak to you and tell you that you are His masterpiece. God doesn't make mistakes; every hair on your head is numbered. Your name is written on the palms of His hands. He delights in you.

It is a wonderful time to separate the fearful diagnosis of cancer to the truthful and life-giving thoughts of God.

We don't want to tip-toe into this important step. We step fully into the abyss of complete trust in God and the glorious realm of Spirit.

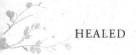

God reassures you. Why? Because He loves you unconditionally and needs you to be a witness to His goodness. He gave you a purpose and that purpose is to do everything for Love. Here's your opportunity.

✳ GRATITUDE

When you do all things mentioned previously, we can't help but have a heart overflowing with love. The body feels gratitude and thanksgiving. It is the life blood of all things good. It raises your thought so high that the body naturally turns on and lights up. Gratitude to God for every little thing is the ticket. Say thank you out loud. Give praise to Love all day in every way. Sing psalms of gratitude and praise for our most gracious God. He didn't cause you to have cancer, but He sure helps you when you most need it. Gratitude healed me and keeps me aligned to this day. It is the ultimate alignment. One can't be in fear and love at the same time, so fill your heart and mind with thanksgiving to Love. A side benefit to giving thanks is that it just feels awesome.

Remember, aligning with divine Love is the most natural way to live. One doesn't have to wait for a major challenge to do it. In fact, the more we practice aligning when life is "good," the easier it will be, and the faster we'll align, when the hard waves of life hit.

Staying in alignment with Source simply means that we are aligned with the way God made us; whole, healthy, happy, and free from anything that is not good. I have found that it is the most effective way to heal not only sickness and disease, but also broken relationships with ourselves and others.

Get ready to embark on a new journey. It will most likely be different from anything you've ever done. The new path is powerful and loving. It means committing to your life, challenges and all, and growing closer to God. You have a choice to make. Are you going to fall apart or rise in the strength of Spirit? Let's roll up our sleeves and do the work now and not wait another day.

chapter 4

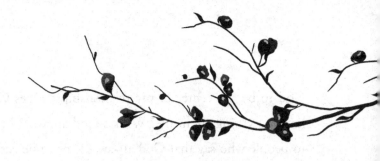

Calm Surrender to Divine Love

What does it mean to surrender to divine Love's will? How many times have you gone to God, begging Him to help you? Instead of begging, have you tried surrendering to the spiritual fact that you are made in His image? What about praying a prayer of affirmation of all the good He has already done? Maybe you can begin your prayer with gratitude?

What happens when fear runs rampant and you can't seem to get a peaceful thought? Pride and self-will once ran the show in my life. I ran ahead of the band, thinking I knew better. It feels so much better to stop and wait on God to lead the way, and that is what I learned to do when going through the ugly, scary claim called cancer.

Ask yourself, where does divine Love live or reside? Can I trust the health of my body to God? Can I trust

God to be the center of my relationships? Does God know anything about me? Who is God anyway? I talk to people who say that God always seems to be across the street. She seems so far away. Clients say, "Yeah, someday I'll take the time to get to know God. I'm really busy right now." I always knew I had a sweet connection to divine Love, but when cancer hit, I was all the way "in." At the moment I was first diagnosed with cancer, I seriously doubted there was a God because I was angry with Him. I wanted to push Him away because I thought He deserted me. I felt that God turned His back on me, so I would turn my back on Him. After I gained my spiritual footing, I realized that God was the one to deliver me from this crisis. I then stepped fully into being an active participant on my healing journey.

WILLINGNESS TO LEARN

One day, while sitting in church, our lay minister read something from the platform. It was a beautiful statement read once a month. To paraphrase, he read that we are not to criticize, judge, or condemn our fellow man. My ears always perk up when that is read because I don't want to be found guilty of doing any of that to family, friends, and even those I don't personally know.

I pondered the words read from the desk and asked God to give me a new understanding of those words. All of a sudden, the other shoe dropped, and I visualized a mirror before my face. It's as if Spirit said, "Yes, Pam, you're pretty good at not doing those things to others, but you are really bad at doing that to yourself."

Yikes. I felt such deep compassion for myself and what I did to malpractice myself, the awesomely fabulous daughter of God. How dare I criticize, judge, or condemn God's daughter, me. After church, I went home, still thinking about this new revelation. I got my dictionary out and looked up the three words. When I got to the word "condemnation," my mouth dropped open, because one of the definitions is "to render oneself incurable."

Whoa. I stopped in my tracks, dropped my head in pure humility, and said, "please forgive me, God, I never meant to condemn one of Your creations, made in Your image. When I criticize, judge, or condemn myself, I do that to God." The interesting thing is that this learning was smack dab in the middle of my cancer journey. I changed my ways immediately and learned to love myself the way God does. It has made all the

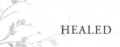

difference in the world how I relate to myself during life's crises. I know to treat myself with the deepest compassion and tender love, forgiving all judgments of myself right away. Forgiveness is one of the major keys to get into alignment with Love. Why? Because God always forgives, and we must, too, in order to be free.

ROY

Roy was diagnosed with cancer of the prostate. He became extremely fearful and immobile. Roy found my name and contact information through a friend who was also a client of mine. We went right to work to see through his fearful thinking. I stood shoulder to shoulder with Roy, coaching him through constant alignment with what was true about him being made in the "image and likeness of God." He indulged in way too much smoking and drinking. He felt God was punishing him because of his lifestyle. I made sure I coached him away from that lie. God loved Roy, and his diagnosis of prostate cancer was simply not His will for one of his precious sons. One of the things I loved about working with Roy was his receptivity to change. He became almost childlike as he dropped his false sense of manhood, bravado and all.

He chose to work with the medical profession while working with me. Our work together gave him tremendous confidence as we eradicated fear and what it tried to do to him. In essence, it tried to kill him.

We discussed what true "manhood" was, because the cancer he was diagnosed with was located in the male reproductive organ. Roy began to see himself as a man of God, purposeful and strong. He understood that he had a job to do and that was to glorify God in everything he did. This new understanding strengthened him and gave him a reason to live.

I recall the same reasoning I had when I went through my cancer journey. My cancer had spread through my reproductive organs and, before I learned to align with how God sees me, I felt I was being punished for perhaps being too codependent and promiscuous with men. I soon learned that that wasn't true about myself as the gorgeous daughter of God. Love always gives us chances to redirect our lives.

We talked about Roy's preciousness in the eyes of God. His cancer treatments went smoothly as he kept his thoughts on what God knew about him. I assured him that he did nothing wrong and was not being punished. I coached him with the understanding that his cancer diagnosis was here for him to learn and grow Spiritward. He took to my coaching like a duck to water. One soon learns, as I did, that there is no time to waste. The lesson is in our face, and we must align with Love totally and completely.

The festering and inflammation in his prostate abated when he learned to forgive himself for all judgment he put on himself and others. In other words, Roy was angry and scared. He was drowning in booze, cigarettes, and junk food. He didn't like himself. I coached Roy in how to love and care for himself in the most honoring way. He understood that taking good care of himself was a way of giving gratitude to God. It opened his thought to new and healthy possibilities. He was incredibly receptive, which is inevitable when one does the work to align with Love.

Roy became more patient. He used Jesus's Sermon on the Mount as an example of how to live and a springboard to living a more aligned life with God.

Roy and I worked for nearly a year together. We built on what was presented and taught to him. There was mental backsliding as fear tried to keep him immobilized, but he persevered. He was dedicated to putting on the new man and changing his ways.

Today, Roy checks in with me when he needs extra help to buoy himself from the fear he feels whenever he feels an ache or pain. Medically speaking, the tumor shrunk, and he is making great progress. Roy has a new lease on life and says he is learning to enjoy God as his ever-present friend and mentor. When I see him now, he stands tall, with his shoulders back and chin raised.

KNOWING WHO GOD IS CHANGES EVERYTHING

While reading this book, you might ask the question, "what do I really know about God, anyway?" Great question. Let me tell you about the God I've grown to know and love. The God I moved into alignment with is pure Love. I can depend on Her. I call on God's angels to protect my children and me. Divine Love is both male and female. I always use the masculine and feminine interchangeably to make the point. He is everywhere. She is filling all space and time. He is the only power of the universe even though it seems like there's many other conflicting forces and powers. She made the whole world, the galaxy we're living in, and the entire universe belongs to God. The God I align with doesn't punish, shame, or guilt His children. His work of creating everything was done in the first chapter of Genesis, so why do we doubt this and make life so difficult by living in lack and low-vibrational thinking? God didn't make flawed thinking, and when we align with divine Love, we think and feel as God does. I love Genesis I and believe in it with my whole heart. Why? Because God's work is finished and complete, and it is "very good."

Genesis II is a wonderful allegory of the human condition, flawed in every way. We all have a choice. Were we made in the image and likeness of God, or were we made from the dust of the ground? When I was healed of cancer and moved into alignment with what God knows about me and the universe, I stayed entirely in the first chapter, so proving I cannot be made in the image and likeness of God (spiritually), *and* also from the dust of the ground as related in the second Chapter of Genesis (materially).

I yielded to Love's will for my life knowing that Her will is good and perfect. It included life to its fullest and a healthy and strong body. I know there are many a doubting Thomas out there, and that's okay. Everybody gets to choose for themselves. I chose to align with the Divine.

THE PRIVILEGE OF
CHOOSING ONE'S THOUGHTS

Another thought to ponder is the idea that we get to choose what thoughts we want to think. In the book, *Man's Search for Meaning* by Viktor Frankl, he writes that everything can be taken from a man except for his ability to think correctly. Frankl was a Holocaust survivor. He witnessed some of the worst brutality on this earth. He knew that everything could be stripped from a person's experience – such as their home, clothes, family members, food and shelter – but the one thing our worst enemy can't take from us is our ability to think.

I knew I could choose love or fear. I felt empowered to choose life or death. I chose to forgive myself and others instead of holding onto resentment and hatred. I learned not to compare my experience to others. This was my curriculum and not anyone else's. Cancer was the perfect challenge for me to ascend higher in my development as a child of God. I learned how to look cancer straight in the eye and say, "I know who you are, you're a liar and a cheat. 'Get thee behind me, Satan.'" I became fearless and ever so courageous. I listened to the voice of Love all day, every day. Every time I'd feel a pain in my body, I knew I had a choice on how I wanted to think about it. I chose, like Viktor Frankl, to be firm with the thoughts I wanted to let into my consciousness. I chose healthy thoughts, not fearful, sick thoughts. I listened to my own heart of love instead of everyone else as the authority of my life. After all, that's how it all started; by looking into my own loving heart where the kingdom of God resides and aligning with what Love knows about me.

BECOMING A WARRIOR FOR GOD

Begin to relate to yourself and every challenge with the heart of a warrior; a warrior for God, for good. Learn how to put your foot squarely on the neck of the serpent. Why? Because as stated in the first chapter of Genesis, you have dominion over anything that is unlike God. You live in the kingdom of God. His work is done; that's already been established. Let that be your starting point, and never allow lack or fear to enter your thinking. You are worth it.

chapter 5

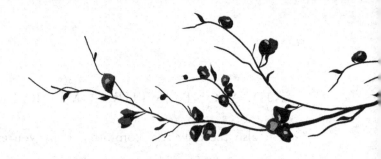

Gratitude Heals

I love to ponder what it means to heal from within. It's self-honoring to know that you have all the answers as you commune with divine Love. The Bible verse from Psalms 139:7-10 illustrates perfectly that there is no place where God is not. "Whither shall I go from thy spirit? or whither shall I flee from thy presence? If I ascend up into heaven, thou art there: if I make my bed in hell, behold, thou art there. If I take the wings of the morning, and dwell in the uttermost parts of the sea; Even there shall thy hand lead me, and thy right hand shall hold me."

How is it possible for God to be everywhere and to be a saving *and* healing presence? Because we live in the consciousness of divine Love. Where God is, we are. What Love knows about is the only opinion that matters.

GOD, ALONE, IS THE COMFORTER

God is also the only true comforter. Have you ever needed to be comforted by a parent, a partner, a teacher, or a friend, and they simply weren't present for you in the way you needed to be comforted? Divine Love is always present, will never leave you comfortless, and delights in comforting you. God is our true Mother and Father.

I AM NOT A VICTIM
OF MY CIRCUMSTANCES

One day, shortly after returning home from the hospital, I was resting upstairs in our bed. I asked my husband to please make our children dinner that night. He said he would. I thanked him and asked if he could bring me a bowl of spaghetti after he fed the kids. He said he would.

I heard rustling downstairs as he was making dinner. The sounds of dishes clanging and energetic kids winding down from the day made me feel so happy. As I lay on the bed, I reached out to divine Love and thanked Her for this moment. It felt so awesome to be feeling a little better again. My family ate an early dinner around

5:30 p.m., and I heard them cleaning the kitchen afterward. Things quieted down as I assumed Colleen and John had started their homework. I thought, "Yay, it is my turn to eat. I'm so hungry." My appetite had fully returned, and I anticipated a big bowl of spaghetti. I knew that my husband would be coming upstairs and into the room to feed me any minute now.

I felt a little puzzled when 6:00 p.m. came and went with no sign of my husband and my dinner. I tried to call to him, but he didn't hear me. I think I heard the news on the television playing.

When the clock turned 7:00 p.m. and then 8:00 p.m., my thoughts turned into sadness that I wasn't noticed. I felt abandoned and worthless. The awful thoughts came to me that I wasn't worth a bowl of spaghetti, no one cares about me, least of all my husband. After feeling like a victim, I got angry and indignant. I knew that, by 9:30 p.m. with no dinner, I had a choice to make on how I wanted to relate to this Pandora's box of feelings I had running in my head. I had felt invisible to Tim my entire married life, and this was just the icing on the cake. Where was my bowl of spaghetti? I was trying to fortify my body, and nobody saw me.

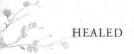

Somewhere between 10:00 and 10:30 p.m., my husband came into the bedroom rather nonchalantly and handed me the bowl of spaghetti I so anxiously awaited. I looked at his face and instantly thought that I had a choice. I could be angry or grateful. Yes, dinner was late. Yes, I was starving. Yes, I felt abandoned, but he remembered. Yes, the dinner was stone-cold, but I decided to look him in the eyes and say, "Thank you so much for this bowl of spaghetti, it looks delicious. Also, thank you for feeding the kids and getting them to bed. I am so grateful," and I meant it.

Why do I share this story? Because it was vitally important to my healing. I had a choice on how to think about this situation, and I chose to use sincere gratitude for my husband instead of anger. Anger equals cancer. It was time for me to change the way I related to him and I did.

chapter 6

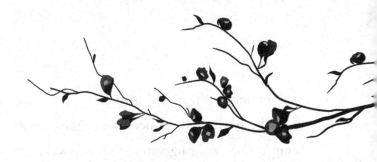

Healing – Divinely Natural and Organic

Dear God, what am I to learn from this life-les-son named cancer? Is this all a sad joke? Did you cause this to happen to me, Spirit? Why would an all-loving God do this to Her child? These were some of the questions I needed to ask myself. I took a lot of time for mental self-examination. I pondered what it meant to "know thyself." If I took responsibility for my poor actions, I could change them to live in accordance and alignment with the way Jesus lived. To have the mind of Christ was my daily prayer.

AN ORGANIC PROCESS

The process of moving into divine Love alignment, I found, was an organic process. It was a yearning to feel good, an exploration of God as the most benevolent force on this earth, and, ultimately, the only true power in the universe. I learned that it wasn't God who brought these challenges to us to "test" us. In fact, that was absurd. If we're all made in the image and likeness of God, then I learned to see through the veil (the lie) of material living, including my body, to the glorious, free-flowing existence called life in God. It was then that I realized that God doesn't send us sickness and disease; She heals it by changing the foundation of our thinking to be in alignment with what She knows about you and me.

I learned how to change my thoughts into alignment with what God knew about me: healthy, purposeful, and here to be a witness to all that God is. I remembered that God's work was done in the first chapter of Genesis. I didn't need to change anything but my thought of who God is, who I am, and what God has already done. In other words, I learned to begin with the truth of all being and not with the problem of poor health and lack. This was a real shift in thought for me.

When I thought about God and all She already did, I grew more and became more grateful. It was effortless. I began to compartmentalize my days. I thought I could certainly give thanks to God for a half-day. A half-day turned into a whole day, and the rest is history. After all, I had much to be grateful for. This wasn't an intellectual process; it was a heart-centered process. Meaning, expressing gratitude wasn't about over-thinking but, instead, it was a healing process in which I moved into alignment and felt God and me as one-emotionally, physically, mentally, and spiritually. I can't help but feel good, and gratitude naturally comes as a by-product of feeling good.

THE BIBLE'S HEALING MESSAGES BECAME MY COMFORTER

I happen to love the spiritual interpretation of the Bible. I resonate with a more enlightened sense of the Bible and not a literal translation. I take Jesus's teachings to heart. I read the Beatitudes and Sermon on the Mount and live by the simple, yet powerful, principles Jesus taught. Many times a day, I practiced the power of stillness and presence. My meditation was on God.

It was at this time that the words from the Psalmist came back to my thought. "I shall not die, but live and declare the works of the Lord." When they first came

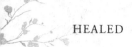

to me in the middle of the night, I felt they were words coming directly from God giving me hope and keeping me buoyed. Now they sounded like gentle marching orders from Love. I talked and wrote about my experience of cancer and aligning with Love. I began a healing practice where people would call me for prayerful support and healing. Women and men called me constantly, looking for something to hold on to. They were desperately seeking healing, and I knew I could offer them hope and fill their hearts while sharing my journey of cancer with them. Coaching my clients helped to change their thoughts and align with Love. Many experienced healing after putting on the "new man" and have gone on to live productive and healthy lives.

I have written a lot about physical healing, but my method of moving into Love alignment is true in relationships, as illustrated in my example with my husband. There is so much talk about PTSD, shock, anxiety, and trauma these days, but what if we could avoid all of that before it happens altogether? Once one experiences the awful, life-sucking effects of PTSD, anxiety, shock, and trauma, it is incredibly difficult to work through because they're imprinted in us.

Sometimes life's challenges feel like a big tidal wave coming toward us. We cower, duck our heads, and hold our breath waiting for the wave to pass, hoping that it doesn't hurt or even kill us. It seems like the waves of life come at a faster pace than ever before, and there is no space between the waves to catch a breath. If we understand that our entire life would be secure and safe if we cultivated constant and continual alignment, every day in every way, then we wouldn't be caught off guard and be taken down so violently. It's no wonder people turn to alcohol, drugs, and food to numb and sedate themselves. Life just hurts way too much sometimes.

The benefits of aligning with Love are better health, peace, freedom of thought, freedom of action, clarity, assuredness, and safety, to name just a few. It's good to work in a preventative way. What do I mean by preventative? It means to move into alignment when we wake up before we put our feet on the floor. It means pausing throughout the day to move into alignment, so we aren't caught off guard. It also means setting an intention before going to sleep for a restful and peaceful sleep, aligned with Love, curled up on the lap of Love.

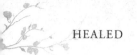

The following are a few alternative phrases for aligning with God that I frequently use:

- The still, small voice within.
- The kingdom of heaven is within.
- We live in the consciousness of divine Love.
- Be still and know that I am God.

Learning that God is closer than the air you breathe establishes the spiritual fact that Love knows you and loves you beyond measure; that challenge or issue is here for you, not to take you down. The problem is here to bring you closer to God and not away from Him. God doesn't bring the problem to you. God delivers you from the problem. God is never testing you. God would never test or tease one of Her precious children, you.

The question comes down to what kind of God do you believe in? Do you understand your worth in the eyes of Love and cherish yourself the way God cherishes you? Do you believe that anything is possible to God? Are you living in the first chapter of Genesis or the second? How can you be made in the image and likeness of God and be made of the dust of the ground? You get to choose.

I happen to love the Adam and Eve story in the second chapter because it's the perfect allegory for the human condition. It's a beautiful juxtaposition and a powerful contrast. Divine Love alignment has never let me down, and its foundation is based fully in 1st Genesis.

MARY

Mary received a cancer diagnosis and remembered seeing an article I had written about how I was healed after all material means and traditional methods had failed. Mary set up an appointment with me, and we talked for an hour. She poured her heart out, relaying all the scary details of what the doctor proposed to her as a plan of action. She was highly emotional as we talked. This was simply a sign that fear ran the show, and we needed to get on top of that. Fear needed to be weeded out of her thoughts before anything else, so we went to work.

We talked about her religious upbringing and what was imprinted in her consciousness as a young child. With my help, Mary began to know God in a whole new way; a totally loving God, never inflicting harm on Her children. She was raised to believe in an anthropomorphic God who judges and punishes

Her children. She never learned that God is Love. I love my coaching clients and how their faces light up when given the opportunity to think about God differently. Mary understood that her parents did the best they could with what they knew about religion and God. She lovingly forgave her parents for raising her in a fear-based religion. She was thirsty to know more about God as Love.

We discussed who she was in the eyes of divine Love; how she was made "in the image and likeness" of God, perfect and whole. This was a refreshingly new way for her to think about herself. We replaced the thought of herself as a "miserable sinner" who was being punished by God with the thought of seeing herself as the "King's daughter, all glorious within." We talked about her genuine worth and priceless presence. I reassured her of her purpose and talked about God's unconditional love for her.

Then we talked about what a cheat and liar fear is. It is the "talking serpent" in the second chapter of Genesis, trying to tempt us from feeling the love of God. The serpent, or fear, tells us we are worthless and unnecessary in God's plan. Aligned with divine Love (what God knows about us), we learn that this is one bald-faced lie, and that fear is just a thought that can be changed in an instant. The practice of becoming immediately aware when fear knocks on the door of consciousness is paramount to stopping it in its tracks. Emphasizing how important the complete eradication of fear is when healing cancer is paramount. Every time fear shows up, look at it straight in the eyes and call it out for what it is – a bald-faced lie about God and man.

This was the first session with Mary. It takes a while for people to understand the vastness of this teaching. We had many more sessions together, allowing truth to sink deeper into her heart while fear left for good. It's the pouring in of love that does the healing. Love washes away all fear. Fear is one of the foundations of disease. It needs to be eradicated from thought.

I held Mary's hand and heart through her cancer journey. She is in a good place now, physically, emotionally, mentally, and spiritually. She feels empowered to go forward in her life with new strength and conviction. Her radiant smile lights up a room.

I am so in love with my coaching clients as they find new meaning in life and become reborn.

chapter 7

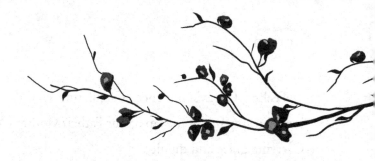

Cancer – Punishment
or Opportunity?

Before we discuss why you are going through this journey called cancer, I want to share a thought process using an acronym for cancer. Sometimes we're afraid of even the word "cancer." The thought of it paralyzes us and makes us shudder. I learned on my cancer journey to stand up to it. As mentioned before, I stood eye-to-eye with it and saw it for what it was: a life stealer, an energy suck, and a sick joke. Part of looking at cancer in the face was relating to it in a new and different way. I took the letters c-a-n-c-e-r and created a method of aligning with divine Love to move into the inner, secret place in my heart where God and I commune as one.

C – Calm surrender to all that God is and what He does for me in the exact moment. Centering myself in my heart of love where all answers reside.

Feeling Christ's presence. Circulating charity and love. Curling up on the lap of our Father/Mother God. Carrying grace and dignity.

A – Aligning with divine Love and allowing myself to be tenderly cared for by God. Relaxing my shoulders while moving into alignment with Spirit as "made in the image and likeness of Love." Allowing the angels to minister messages of love and healing. Allegiance to God's will.

N – Nowness and Nearness– feeling Love's enormous presence filling all space and being the only true power of my life and the universe. The natural process of letting go and letting God.

C – Clarity of purpose and reason for living. Courage to move forward with my hand in God's. What is my purpose? To give glory, gratitude, and thanks to God in everything I do. Canceling any thought opposed to what is true about God and you. Changing my life by putting on the "new man" in accordance with Jesus Christ's example.

E – Exercising my God-given dominion over cancer and the fear that continued to come to mind with every ache and pain. God didn't make it so I don't have to have it. Why? Because God is good and doesn't bring disease into people's lives. It's what we do to ourselves. Extricating fear and its awful effect on my body. Examining my thought to be in alignment with the one Mind, called God. Exhilarating, heartfelt gratitude. Extra special care of myself and my body, the temple of God.

R – Remission. Not your traditional, cancer-related kind of remission, but instead the remission of thoughts and actions that don't serve our highest good and don't glorify God. Remembering who you are and how God made you-perfect, whole, and free. Recommit oneself every day to serving Love. Retract any hurtful and damaging acts or words I have directed at anyone. Rehearse only words of love.

ASK YOURSELF, ARE YOU MAL-ALIGNED WITH GOD?

See how I took the word cancer, looked it straight in the eye, identified what it was trying to do to me, then replaced it with the healing truth? The word cancer or malignancy becomes a little less scary. After all, the word malignancy means "mal-aligned" or badly aligned. If one is badly aligned, then what is he or she badly aligned with? With a lie about you, that's what

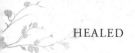
we're aligned with. It means we're wrongfully aligned with something that is not true about you and the way God made you and maintains you. Remember, He is the only power and presence of the universe. The proper alignment then would be divine Love alignment. The Bible eloquently writes, "Ye shall know the truth, and the truth shall make you free." This is the truth as I know it today and, in addition to healing cancer, this truth has helped me in countless ways in working with both myself and others.

OBSERVE, DON'T ABSORB

Daily, I prayed to know what God had in store for me besides being a mother to my two amazing children. I asked Spirit to make the words "Ye shall not die, but live and declare the works of the Lord" known to me so I could carry out my life's purpose in the way Love had intended. As I talked to God, I asked that She strengthen my spiritual core so I could withstand all the hurtful, human stuff that we have to deal with.

I consider myself extremely sensitive and highly empathic. I seem to pick up every emotion from everyone around me. Being in large crowds is unnerving for me. I'm like a psychic sponge that needs lots of downtime to regroup, re-center myself, and readjust my energy. That said, when I know I'll be around a lot of people, I practice getting and staying in alignment. I don't need as much alone time and don't isolate myself like I used to.

As mentioned earlier, I use more proactive and preventative measures when I know I'm going to be with a lot of people for an extended period. I simply take care of myself instead of looking for other people to understand me and maybe take some of my scary feelings away for me. In the past, I looked to my partnerships with men to take away my pain. I see that that was codependency at its finest. I thought my partners knew better than me, and that I was incredibly flawed. I continually looked outside myself for answers which caused an incredible amount of emotional pain. No person on earth can be your "everything." That is just too much pressure to put on anyone. Coming back to myself was the most freeing and exciting thing I've ever experienced. Knowing that no one can give me the time, attention, and love that I crave more than myself. When I write "myself," I speak of my oneness with Love. She is my best friend, my constant companion, my forever partner, and my true Mother and Father who love me unconditionally.

The Bible writes, "Whatever you do, do all to the glory of God." People are so busy trying to find out what their lives' purposes are. They are putting the cart before the horse. When we put God first in everything we do and only want to serve and glorify Her, we will be in the right mindset to hear Love and be guided to the right position or career. If we don't put God first, we just might be spinning our wheels over and over again and getting nowhere or have to backtrack. Aligning with Love first saves a lot of time and heartache.

GOD, HELP ME TO PAY FORWARD THIS HEALING IN SERVICE TO YOU

Another way to repay God for all She has done is to pay forward your learning with others that are going through the same stuff you went through and prevailed. We need each other. We need to see and hear success stories of how people overcame devastating challenges. We need a tender heart and helping hand from those that have walked over the hot coals in their lives and became better people because of it.

We also need to speak words of love to ourselves. Stop punishing yourself. Stop berating yourself. Start embracing your gorgeous self and cherishing your individuality. When we do this, the body softens, and we are less rigid. We can then make decisions aligned with Spirit for the highest good instead of a place of tenseness and rigidity.

LIFE PURPOSE AND RE-MISSION

Since we're talking about cancer it is important to mention the word remission. Again, people get anxious about that word and so fearful that remission of cancer can mean that it's dormant for a while but can come back anytime. That is so scary. When I looked cancer in the eye, I also looked at the word remission. I redefined it in spiritual terms. I took control of my thinking and asked Love what I needed to know. The following is how I use the word, in relation to cancer:

- The cancellation, suspension, and revocation of anything that is not from God.
- A respite, lessening, abatement, easing, decrease, reduction of any thought or action that is not in alignment with divine Love.

81

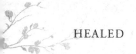

I used the word to mean the remission of sin. I radically turned to God and thought of all the ways I had sinned. I need to forgive myself and others for all judgments. I dug in to excavate wrong, sinful thinking. I emptied the old wine from the vessel of my mind in order to put new wine into my clean, clear vessel of God's creating. I was being born again.

chapter 8

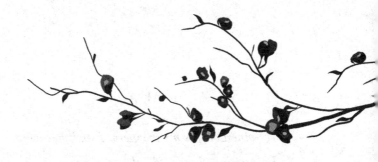

Allowing Divine Love
to Lead

B y now, you know you can access all answers to your questions because you are one with God. You understand how infinitely loved you are and that nothing is too hard for God. You have dropped the notion that you have to be perfect to earn God's love. You've let go of any sense of human perfectionism and see yourself as unapologetically, divinely perfect. Wouldn't all of this suggest to you that you have dominion? Don't you feel stronger now and more aligned? Doesn't this give you immense hope and satisfaction that you can get through this challenge and come out the other end healed?

I love Mary Baker Eddy's interpretation of the 23rd Psalm. She is the discoverer and founder of the Christian Science religion. This particular citation is from her book, *Science and Health with Key the Scriptures.*

PSALM 23

[Divine Love] is my shepherd; I shall not want.
[Love] maketh me to lie down in green pastures:
[Love] leadeth me beside the still waters.
[Love] restoreth my soul [spiritual sense]: [Love] leadeth
Me in the paths of righteousness for His name's sake.
Yea, though I walk through the valley of the shadow of
death, I will fear no evil: for [Love] is with me;
[Love's] Rod and [Love's] staff they comfort me.
[Love] prepareth a table before me in the presence of
Mine enemies: [Love] anointeth my head with oil;
My cup runneth over.
Surely goodness and mercy shall follow me all the days of
my life; And I will dwell in the house [the consciousness]
Of [Love] forever.

Let's break this Psalm down. Eddy uses the name divine Love or Love for God. Love is our way-shower and shepherd. In other words, God directs us to the right direction to take in life. If we feel lost, He shows us the right way to go. If we are fearful, He will shepherd us out of danger to a safe place. Ultimately, we don't want or wish for anything else but to be guided by God. Please think about this in relation to your cancer journey. This will ground and strengthen you. It will offer so much confidence and keep you on track.

Divine Love causes us to lie down in green pastures. Those pastures are a soft place for us to lay our heads. They are a cool, still place filled with peace. Divine Love leads us to still waters. We know that sheep will not drink from turbulent waters. Love is providing us, as His beloved sheep/children, calm, still waters where we can drink without fear and chaos.

Love restores my spiritual sense. There aren't any other senses. The spiritual is the real; the material is unreal. The spiritual heals, the material perpetuates the dream of sickness. Love leads all on the right path and makes no mistakes. We do this to glorify God and give all honor and glory to Him alone.

THE VALLEY AND DEPRESSION

The valley of death is simply a low, depressed state of consciousness. It is where we feel frightened and lost. The shadow is just that – a shadow. It's not real. It's a suggestion that death is real and that the thought of it wants to "shadow" or cloud our thinking to make us fearful and feel like there is no use in trying. It's a dark,

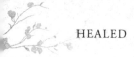

ominous shadow. One thinks they'll never get through that valley, but with God as their shepherd, they will surely get through with dominion and strength. We learn that we don't have to fear evil (cancer) because God is right there with us in that scary valley giving us all the confidence we need. God wants us to succeed and experience a victory in the school of life, and this is our present curriculum. He would never give us something too hard or impossible to do. Love's rod gently prods us along the path out of the valley just like a true shepherd. Love's staff is there for us to lean on as we pass through the valley laden with craggy rocks and lurking animals. Just think about how God is providing for us during this valley experience named cancer. He continues to comfort us in our darkest hour.

ENEMIES ARE SIMPLY THOUGHTS THAT DON'T COME FROM GOD

Divine Love prepares a table for us in the presence of our enemies. Who and what are our enemies? Could our enemies be fear, depression, exhaustion, weakness, and the overwhelming desire to throw in the towel and give up? Love anoints my head with oil – how cool. Doesn't this represent the fact that we are chosen by

God and anointed as His chosen? That He has put His stamp of approval on our foreheads?

When we are grateful for all that God is lovingly doing for us, then we are grateful beyond measure. My cup runneth over means that we can't begin to contain all the good that God is giving us. It is spilling over onto the saucer.

God's mercy and goodness follow us all day, every day. There is no escaping that. Lastly, what does it mean to dwell in the house of the Lord? Eddy explains it as dwelling in the consciousness of Love. To me, it means that we are a perfect and complete idea of God, perfectly made and maintained. In other words, we hang out as Love's ideas. This spiritual fact is unchangeable, permanent, and intact. We couldn't leave if we wanted to. God's house represents God's consciousness; a perfect state of being where we are safe and sound.

I share the 23rd Psalm because it was deeply healing for me as I went through the valley I call cancer. It kept me feeling buoyed and uplifted. My mind felt at peace when I pondered the words from this healing Psalm. It gave me hope and assurance that the valley was a temporary state of being and that, with God, I could get through this wilderness state I call the valley.

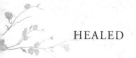

HEALING PROMISES FROM GOD

Friends, the Bible is chock-full of promises, assuring us of God's full presence in times of trouble. During my cancer struggle, I allowed Spirit to talk to me through Scripture. I embodied many favorite passages and clung to them like a mother clutching her baby in the darkest of storms. I would not let go because they gave life. My ship (body) was battered, but it kept afloat with tattered sails until the ocean became calm and the wind ceased. God was at the helm of my ship, captaining with precision. My battle cry was "thank you, God, I trust in you to keep me safe and alive. Thank you, God."

VICTIM MENTALITY OR VICTORIOUS?

Do you believe you have a choice of how you relate to your cancer diagnosis? I hope after reading this chapter, you have an infinite amount of hope. Think, for a moment, that you can relate to cancer with dignity and grace. Think of it as an opportunity to advance in your earth's curriculum (your learning). Cherish the thought of helping others on their cancer journeys because you've experienced what they're going through. The scripture writes, "Hope thou in God." I found I didn't have a choice but to fully hope in God and follow Him in all ways. Before my healing came, I was told I had a short time to live. I was faced with my mortality. After aligning with divine Love and immersing myself in scripture and feeling Love running through me, as me, I was able to step into the abyss of unknowing. Love caught me mid-leap, placed me on solid ground, and showed me the way through the valley of despair. When all was said and done, I wouldn't have missed this opportunity for the world because of what I learned, and now have the golden privilege of sharing my healing with the world.

"Thank you, dear God. I am forever indebted to you. Please show me how I can best serve You." Amen and so it is.

chapter 9

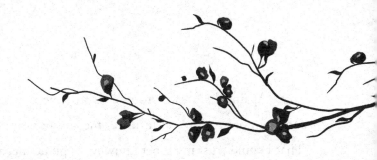

God and Me –
the Perfect Team

By now you know that my method of aligning with divine Love is not a traditional method of healing. Yes, I went the medical route and don't regret a moment of it because of all the angels in disguise I met along the way and the deep caring love I experienced in hospitals and medical facilities. Every time I was told that there was no guarantee I would survive, I fell apart for while only to get back up with a vengeance. Let me tell you what that looked like.

As always, my Bible was a constant source of strength. Citations would come to my thought throughout the day and night, which I interpreted as God speaking to me and giving me the spiritual sustenance I needed to keep going and keep fear at bay. One favorite is, "God in the midst of thee is mighty. He will save." Again, this was a promise that divine Love, the kingdom of heaven, was inside of me and not outside. That I could trust my inner knowing to guide me, and that God is saving me in the present moment. This coupled with my new duty and privilege to glorify God in everything I do filled me with immense light. Speaking of light, I learned to lighten up. In other words, to live in the light, God's light. That is true alignment. Aligned with the light of Love whenever and wherever I was. "Let your light so shine before men that they may see your good works and glorify God in heaven."

I became reclusive because I couldn't control other people's experience of me, and it was too much effort. I needed to save my energy for my children and their needs. My children and I had a routine. They didn't know that I had cancer until years later because I didn't want to burden them and cause them to be fearful for their mommy's life. I would pick them up from school, feed them a snack, have a little playtime, then dinner, homework, baths, bedtime stories then lights out. When they were asleep, I would go downstairs and pace the floor making great demands on divine Love to show me the way. Speaking out loud I would say, "tell me what I need to know, God. I need you, show me how to live, I want to live to raise my children." I cried, screamed into pillows, crumbled to my knees begging God to save me. I didn't care if my husband heard me. He isolated himself during times I was unhinged. I guess I was just too much for him.

My world had become weighty. I took everything seriously, and I felt that I carried the weight of the world on my shoulders. I felt I was solely responsible for the care of my children. I felt it was my job to make sure that Colleen and John were academically grounded and even thriving. They had to have cute clothes, the right hairstyles, be on the best sports teams, and the list goes on. I thought I had to be a perfect woman. I had to cook perfect, nutritious meals, furnish a gorgeous home and keep it spotless. It was my job to make my husband happy at the cost of my happiness. I felt if everyone else was happy, then I would be happy. I had to look perfect, act perfect, present myself and my family to the world perfectly. Be the perfect church member, never make a mistake, be a perfect, caring daughter to my parents, and a perfect sister to my siblings. I just couldn't get a break, and then I received the cancer diagnosis. When I received the phone call that my test results were back and that I needed immediate

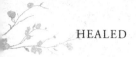

surgery my veneer began to crack-my perfectly coiffed hair and makeup were not going to save my life. Life as I knew it was over, and I needed to find a new way of being. Things needed to change, fast.

How could I be different than whom I knew myself to be? Where do I begin? Where was that confident flight attendant of days gone by? What happened to the bubbly young girl who found excitement in everything? My light had dwindled to a flickering flame ready to be snuffed out at any moment with cancer.

The simple fact was that I was still alive and breathing. I had the opportunity to change my thoughts and actions and get going with all the learning I came to earth to do.

THE CONFERENCE ROOM

I have a funny way of thinking about what happens before and after we incarnate to our "next experience." For me, my next experience was to be spent on the planet Earth, so there I was. Just suppose for a moment that before we incarnated, we met with whomever (I'll call them "the elders") in the heavenly conference room. They said, "Pam, what would you like to accomplish on Earth this time around? What issues would you like to work on? Patience, gentleness, more love for yourself? Do you want to help the environment, animals, children, the elderly, women's rights?" They told me that I could do anything to better the world, but I must put God first in everything I do. The elders also said that I might forget around the age of five what my purpose was, and that there's a good chance the world's problems might seem too much to handle. They said that life would be perfectly set up for me to learn my lessons, and it was.

THE WEIGHTINESS OF
EARTHLY THINKING

Life before cancer was about looking for love in all the wrong places, trusting other people more than trusting myself, not trusting Life/God, thinking I had to do everything or it wouldn't get done, thinking I had to be perfect to be loved, and feeling my family and home had to be the model for all to admire. I fell short of all of the above, and I got sick with cancer. My body felt the extreme resentment I had for my husband because of our financial situation, his lack of attention toward me, his emotional absence as a father, and on and on and on.

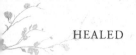
It is simply a story about a broken woman, crying out for help until she turned wholeheartedly to God, stepped into an abyss of the unknown, and surrendered to God. I was a tired, sad, and angry woman until I wasn't – pure and simple. I had nowhere to go but to the arms of Love, and that I did, entirely and completely. I became a God-pleaser and dropped the people-pleasing. I allowed my genuine beauty and light to shine through me naturally and didn't require makeup to make me more beautiful than God had already made me.

Another amazing thing about moving into divine Love alignment is that it doesn't cost a dime. We can do this anywhere we find ourselves. It can be used for every human issue and challenge we find ourselves in. Conflict in relationships, challenges with children, business and church meetings, and even a better relationship with yourself is benefited and healed by moving into alignment with what God knows about all of it. Ultimately, one learns that glorifying God and moving into alignment are the same. In the end, we learn that it is only God that will truly make us happy. People will come and go from your life through break-ups, divorces, and death. Friends will be there, sometimes, but not all the time. Children will grow up and make a life of their own. What's left? God and you. Yep, that's it, just you and God. And, by the way, that is enough.

chapter 10

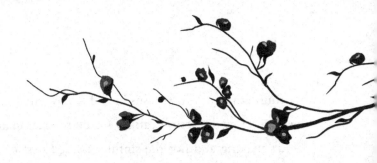

Commitment, Dedication, and Perseverance

Are you ready to hop onto the path of healing? Have other means and methods of healing fallen short of their promises? Are you ready to be "all-in" and fully committed to being the vibrant and healthy person God created? Divine Love alignment was the missing ticket for me. There's nothing wrong with salt baths, crystals, meditation, hands-on healing, traditional and nontraditional doctors, mud baths, shamans, herbs and chanting, but the one thing that finally worked for me was finding an answer to the question, "who is God and who am I?" Surrendering to Love, trusting Spirit, doing the will of God, understanding I am made in the exact image of God, having the same substance as Her, saved my life.

I learned that, without a shadow of a doubt, this is how Jesus healed and, by the way, scripture writes that we must emulate Christ Jesus in all his ways, including healing. How did Jesus heal? By seeing the real man of God's making and not the sinful, diseased part of the human experience. He separated the sin from the sinner, so to speak, and witnessed only what God made. I gave it a try and was blessed abundantly.

I'M JUST A WOMAN
TRYING TO FIGURE IT OUT

I'm just a woman who decided to follow the breadcrumbs that God placed before my feet; I followed them even though my feet bled and blistered. I kept going with my eye on the prize. Gratitude to God was my staff and rod. Isn't it time to roll up your sleeves and do the work you came here to do? Why do you want to find yourself in that "conference room" again having not done the work that is right under your nose to do now? Scripture writes, "now is the accepted time, behold, now is the day of salvation." My understanding is, why put off the things we need to do today? After all, today is filled with blessings, and it all begins with thought.

I used to think I needed to clean up my past before I could live in the moment. I thought I had to forgive my father before I could have the mindset to heal myself. I thought I needed more degrees and letters behind my name to be worthy. I thought I needed to earn Spirit's love in order to be heard. You get the picture. We need to stop that kind of thinking and get into divine Love alignment immediately, and then we need to stay there. The little gremlin that sits on your shoulder trying to tell you that you are a miserable sinner and that you're nothing is only negative thought and nothing else. It's the serpent in the second chapter of Genesis filling you with fear and self-loathing that needs to be squelched. Know your worth.

DON'T GO ON A WITCH HUNT – FLOW NATURALLY WITH DIVINE LOVE

I wrote of the "remission of sins," but you don't have to go on a witch hunt to try to clean up your whole life before you move into Love alignment. Aligning is free-flowing and organic. In other words, if something or someone comes to mind, and you have a judgment about them, then it is the time to forgive yourself and others. Do it at the moment that person comes to mind, and you're triggered by them. Forgive them of all judgments you have held against them. What an awe-

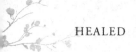

some thought, to know you can move into alignment with Love AND be in remission. That we can empty the old ways of thinking while we are allowing Love to pour in the "new wine" or new, better thoughts.

Picture divine Love alignment as a beautiful brass scale. On one side of the scale is the absolute truth of God and you. In other words, it's what is already true regarding who God is and who you are in God's eyes - perfect, whole, and free. On the other side of the scale is our Earth's schooling, including all our challenges, issues, and problems. They are here for us to learn and grow into the person you wanted to become when you talked with your elders in the conference room. Remember?

HUMAN DAD OR DIVINE HEAVENLY FATHER?

Let me offer an example of how I did this. Shortly after being home from my cancer surgery, I felt I was well enough to host the Easter brunch at my home. I did this almost every year, so it wasn't anything new. I put the call out to family members to bring a favorite dish and to come over for a fun family afternoon of good food and hunting Easter eggs. Everyone responded with a "yes" except my dad. I thought that was odd, so I called him a couple times more until one day, shortly before the gathering, I received a three by five card in the mail which read, "I won't be able to make it to your Easter party, 'Dad.'" I thought that was odd, but the party planning continued.

After Easter, I tried to call him to ask if he was okay, and if I could do anything for him but received no answer. By this time, I felt hurt. I couldn't understand what I did wrong to make him act this way. I was ready to apologize to him and to make amends, but I simply couldn't figure out what I did to make him act this way. I felt depressed and sad because I needed my father. I was barely on the road to recovery and needed all the love I could get. I was afraid and confused. My children needed "Grumpy Gramps," as well. They loved him, but were too young to understand why he didn't show up like he used to. I was at a loss as to what to tell them. My dad stopped talking to me one day – until one day turned into six years.

What happened during those six years? I continued to heal, and Colleen and John continued to grow. As a family, we'd hop in the van and take trips. We'd drive up the coast of California making stops along the way

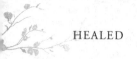

at our favorite towns, laughing and creating memories. Dad lived about an hour and a half north of us. Every single time we'd drive by on the freeway I'd make a call to him which went something like this: "Hi Dad, this is Pam, the kids and I are going to stop at the Apple Farm for dinner just up the road from you. We'll be there at 6:00 p.m., I hope you can make it because we'd love to see you. I love you, Dad." He always screened his calls (you remember answering machines) and would hear my voice and intentionally not pick up the phone on his end. Obviously, he never showed up to meet with us.

For the first year, I would ask my Dad what I did wrong. During the second year, I quit asking. The third year I talked to his answering machine like I was writing in my diary or journal. I told him what the kids were up to, about our new move to the Santa Ynez Valley, our home and our animals. Always, I ended my phone call with, "I love you, Dad."

One might ask me why I was so nice and accommodating. Another might call me a fool for hanging in there. But I knew I had a choice on how to relate to this challenging situation with my dad. It was important for me to use this experience as part of my school curriculum. I knew that it was one, big, awesome opportunity to think of myself, the situation, and my dad differently. Every time I felt like a worthless and awful person, I moved into alignment with Love, my true parent.

I learned how to comfort my own aching heart, having oodles of compassion for the young "Pammy" who just wanted to be loved. I got clear that my dad's actions had nothing to do with who I was as God's cherished daughter. In other words, my dad's lack of communication could not define who I was. Only Love could do that. Believe me, I waffled a lot. I was grounded one moment and completely off-kilter the next. But I was getting stronger every day because I was drawing closer to God, my true Father, and forgiving my earthly dad's actions more and more, quicker and quicker.

I only called him a couple of times in the last year of him not talking to me. Again, "Hi Dad, this is Pam, I love you."

A DAD AND DAUGHTER HEALING

Then, my dad called. I picked up my phone and heard his words, "Hi honey, this is your dad. I'm at the local Santa Ynez Valley airport. Why don't you come by and say hi?" I drove my car like a bat out of hell to the airport where he was standing with his little airplane. We hugged like we always did. He mindlessly chatted about his flying experiences then said, "Well, the wind is picking up, I gotta go." Then he was off into the wild, blue yonder, just like that.

My life continued at home. I didn't tell my kids that I saw Grumpy Gramps. They wouldn't understand. Two weeks later my dad called me again and said, "Hey sweetums, how about meeting me for breakfast?"

I said, "Sure Dad, let me get the kids to school and I'll be right over."

Feeling still numb, I drove to the restaurant, hugged my dad, and sat down to order. I knew I needed to say something for my sanity.

I said, "Hey Dad, you left me in a dark time of my life. I was just starting to heal from cancer, I needed you,, and you abandoned me, what was that about?"

He never looked at me but, instead, stared out the window and changed the subject. Small talk continued, and then the waiter brought us the check. What happened next was the pivotal moment in our relationship. Dad walked me to my car in the parking lot. By now, I knew I needed to say something to him to put an "amen" to our years of not talking. I needed to show up as a complete and whole-souled woman and speak up.

I looked my dad straight in the eyes and said, "Dad, I forgive you, and I love you." No more than a half a second passed, he fell into my arms and bawled like a baby. I held him in my strong arms while he had his moment. I had already forgiven him as I, daily, had moved into alignment with divine Love since the time he stopped talking to me, to be comforted as a true and loving father would. My real Father, God, loves me unconditionally, and He would never abandon me. I needed this lesson. I am grateful for the lesson. I wouldn't have missed it for the world.

After that moment in the parking lot, my Dad called me every day to say he loved me and was so proud of me. From Scripture, "God will restore to us the years that the locust hath eaten." This was certainly a promise that God delivered on because we had a fabulous, loving relationship to the day he died. Divine Love alignment works. It's a tried and true method.

chapter 11

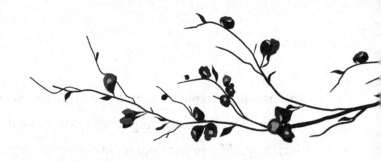

Let's Do This

Here we are, standing on holy ground – on the precipice of something life-changing, yet divinely natural. It takes courage to be human, but the rewards of living in the kingdom of God are no less than a miracle and you can do that here and now. Do you feel the "divine energies of Spirit, bringing you into newness of life?" Divine Love alignment is a way of life. It stops fear and suffering in its tracks. I tried every material remedy to heal cancer and wasn't getting any better until I instinctually surrendered to God and followed Her with my whole heart. The veil lifted off of my emotional and physical pain and fear, so completely that I experienced a brand-new life.

I got to watch my children grow and participate in all their activities. Their "new" mom found ways of not needing to be humanly perfect anymore because perfectionism nearly killed her. God placed me in situations where I could serve Her and use my talents to glorify Her. I learned to give all credit to God for everything. My prayer looked like simple, ongoing chats with divine Love. I learned how to do everything with love. I thank God in the smallest of ways.

When I drive, I drive for God. When I do the dishes, I do them for Her. When my clients and I talk, I do my best to see them as God sees them. Many times, I don't see a human face, but instead, the face of God. It is a gorgeous way to live, and it's here for you, too.

We spend so much time being disillusioned by worldly problems. That's because we start with the idea of "lack." But God didn't make lack. He doesn't cause a lack of health, finances, resources, ideas, etc. Divine Love alignment begs us to see and know what God knows.

Remember Genesis 1? "He made everything and behold it was very good." There is no lack in the words "very good."

It's time to wake up and live in the light. Do the work now. It's nothing short of life-giving.

I am here to hold your hand and guide you. Don't wait. I am here to witness your true essence. Most of all, I am here to be a mirror for you so you can do this same work and advance your soul in the classroom of life. Ponder the word ascension. Look it up in your dictionary. Embody the meaning, and then you will know your real purpose for being on this earth.

I'll leave you with just one more story on how I aligned with divine Love during one of the most critical moments in my life.

GOD, THE ONLY POWER AND PRESENCE

While working for American Airlines as a flight attendant, I took a number of months off from flying and was hired to teach emergency procedural training to the flight attendants at my home base, San Francisco. This was done in the evenings in one of the airplane hangars in a mock-up. I was one member on a team of five people who taught every night.

After teaching I would return to my downtown San Francisco flat late each night. One night after hours of being at work and getting ready for bed, I opened my bedroom door to go to the kitchen to get a glass of water and was confronted by a man, crouched on my hallway floor. As the light from my room shone on him, I screamed three times. The roommate I shared

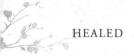

a room with was away on a business trip. My other roommate was a few feet away, sleeping in her room with the door shut. The man jumped on me, covered my face with a pillowcase, and put me onto the floor of my bedroom, face down. My roommate didn't hear my screams for help and never woke up.

I was paralyzed with fear. I've heard it said that in a crisis like that, one either fights for their life or becomes lifeless. I became as lifeless as a wet noodle. I had no fight in me. As I was lying face down on the cold hardwood floor, I knew I was completely helpless. I had no one to save me, no one to rescue me. I was lost.

The man seemed nervous. He was anxious and the energy in the room was intensely fearful and frantic. My purse was a couple of feet from me in a chair. It was then I realized he wasn't there for my purse; he was there to rape me.

Many years later, while working through "women's issues" related to cancer in my reproductive organs, the rape incident came to mind. I had read that the act of raping means that "women have to bend over and take it." This was startling for me. I began to heal and have a healthy and vibrant sense of what it means to be a woman after aligning with God's thought of women and what they represent. All these situations were a tremendous opportunity to understand and feel God's presence and power in the most life-threatening situations.

NOW BACK TO MY STORY

The man raised my flannel nightgown to my mid-back. I felt the blade of a cold knife brushing against my skin. I reached out to God with my whole heart. I had nowhere to go but within. I was deathly afraid. At this time, I felt a powerful shift in the room. I felt the presence of Love, which is the only way I can explain it. It filled the room and I felt enormous peace after feeling fierce fear. As I turned inward and focused on God, I talked to the man.

I said, "You are a good man and you don't have to do this. God loves you and doesn't want you to hurt me. You are God's man. He loves you."

The man got angry and said, "shut up or I'm going to hurt you." But I couldn't stop talking. The words flowed out of me. I repeated the words, "you are a good man and God doesn't want you to hurt me."

He pressed the knife a little harder on my back and told me to shut up, or he was going to hurt me badly.

I persisted. It was a power and force coming out of me that simply wouldn't stop. He asked me if my roommate was home. He had been watching my roommates and me closely. I said I wasn't sure.

The man pulled me up off the floor, walked me to my roommate's door, pulled the pillowcase off my head and threw me on the floor. As I jumped on my roommate's bed, she woke up. I grabbed her as I opened the window by her bed. We lived on the second floor, but I told her to get ready and that we were going to jump.

The man ran out of the room as I yelled out the window, "help, help, rape, rape." I thought he was going to get his knife but come to find out he ran down the stairs and out the front door taking a set of our keys with him. Neighbors ran up the stairs and into our apartment with bats and knives ready for battle. We called the police to report what happened. They arrived and it was a long night of having to rehearse what happened. Everyone left and I was alone with my thoughts. I realized that I had naturally moved into divine Love alignment to access God as the only power and presence of the universe and present to save me. I can't help but think that the man that broke into my home to rape me felt the same.

Had anyone in his life ever told him that he was a good man, God's man? I believe that he was saved that night as well. I sure hope so.

FROM MY HEART TO YOURS

Why do I write about this dramatic story in a book about my healing of cancer? Because this is a theme in my life. I want to share the one thing that heals above all others; the power of prayer and turning fully to divine Love. I have much more to share about how I aligned with divine Love to heal. It's time to ask, how can I be of service? How can I help you align with divine Love and heal?

chapter 12

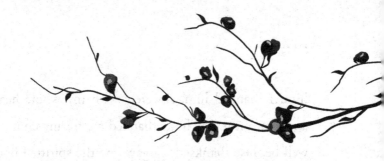

Conclusion

My wish for you is radiant health and a mind aligned with the mind of God. This sounds like a tall order, but it's possible right here and now. I want you to know and understand that aligning with divine Love is the one thing that will bring peace of mind while you place all your cares and worries on God. It is the highest form of meditation as we listen to the thoughts of God and not everyone else or meditate with a blank mind.

In this book, you learned what "aligning with divine Love" looks and feels like. You have read my personal story of aligning when every single material remedy failed to work. I loved adding my story of how gratitude is a major component to healing when my husband brought me a cold bowl of spaghetti four hours after everyone else ate, and I had a choice on how I wanted to relate to it. My choice was to berate him or thank him. I thanked him, sincerely with my whole heart, and I meant it. My body thanked me for my choice as well because thanksgiving gave me the spiritual boost and nourishment I needed so badly at that time.

In this book, I wrote about how forgiveness of my dad, at a time that he stopped communicating with me for six years, proved to be the most wonderful spiritual lesson, because I learned who my true father and mother was. I was able to forgive my earthly dad for his behavior and all the judgments I had on him. I learned how to parent myself and see that I am enough. What ensued after our reconciliation was nothing short of a miracle. Unconditional love for each other ensued, and we talked every single day until the day he died.

I had no idea if I was going to live or die when going through the dark valley of fear. I used every remedy and called every healer I knew for help to no avail, until I found all the answers within my own heart. I hope, dear reader, I have emphasized the spiritual fact that you have a heavenly host of angelic helpers at your side at all times. Don't be afraid to ask for help. The angels are ready and willing to deliver you from the depths of despair anytime you ask. How do I know this? Because

I proved this for myself in one of the most crucial times of my life.

When the rapist broke into my apartment in San Francisco, I immediately aligned with the powerful presence of God, and all I could do was speak the truth to this man. He was a good man, doing a bad thing. Divine Love was present for both of us, and we were both delivered from experiencing something awful; me being raped, him doing the raping.

I couldn't keep the secrets to aligning with God to myself anymore and wanted to share this healing path for everyone going through a cancer diagnosis, a difficult marriage, raising a family, and low self-esteem.

My hope is that you'll feel encouraged to give aligning with divine Love a try. You have free will to do whatever inspires you. Choose the highest and most "right" thing to do for you.

I found the inspired word of the Bible incredibly helpful, so I chose to openly share the passages that kept me on a straight and narrow path. Certain citations in the Bible became illuminated and seemed to jump off the page when I needed them most. I felt the warmth of each word as a wink and promise from God that continues to carry me to this day.

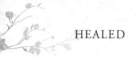

Let's suppose you took the intended meaning of my book and applied it to your life. What would that look like? The client stories I shared are wonderful examples of changed and upgraded lives after aligning with God. Health was restored. Marriages were saved. Self-confidence and self-worth were salvaged. Clients became less dependent on popular opinion and more trusting in what Love is saying.

I have seen my clients become gentler people and less judgmental. Readers will understand after reading this book that fear is at the basis of all human discord, including all disease, and that they have dominion over anything that is not from God.

I trust you will feel a shift in thought while reading my book, giving you immense sense of hopefulness.

I love my clients. Each one keeps in close touch with me, knowing that I am here for them if they feel stuck in the process. Clients have used words like "the most palpable love they've ever know," "a warmth bath," "a space where time stood still, and all there was was love," and "a soft feeling of pure knowing" to describe the simple process of aligning with divine Love. They have shared how aligning has become more natural and their "go-to" place for healing.

I am incredibly grateful to God that I listened to Her and wrote this book. My intention is to help as many people by giving them hope after reading my story of overcoming cancer. It is with a servant's heart that I offer these pages of hope and healing.

God abundantly loves you. My prayer is that you feel this life-saving truth and live an aligned life with Love.

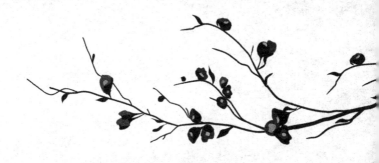

Acknowledgments

Thank you to Angela Lauria and
The Author Incubator's team for helping me
bring this book to print.

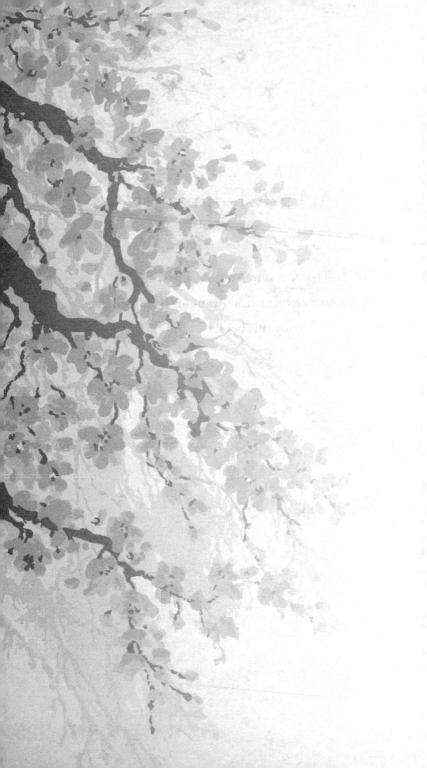

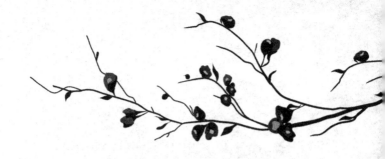

Thank You

Thank you to all of you who took the time to read my book, *Healed: A Divinely Inspired Path to Overcoming Cancer*. Your health and happiness mean the world to me.

I trust you are now amply inspired to cultivate your own unique relationship with divine Love. I would have been so grateful if I had someone to hold my hand and heart when I went through my own journey of cancer – a guide along the trail to encourage and strengthen me. I have helped many people find their way to the heart of Love and find their way past fear and doubt.

As a thank you for reading my book, I'd like to offer you a complimentary, twenty-minute session to see if we're a good fit. Hop onto my website http://www.PamelaHerzer.com/ and schedule time on my calendar. While you're there, sign up for my free newsletter. I care about you. My intention is for you to heal and live an abundant life, giving gratitude to God for everything. Let's do this!

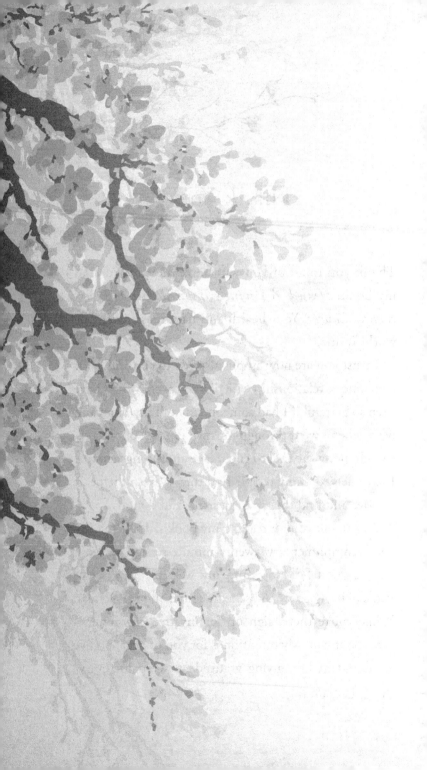

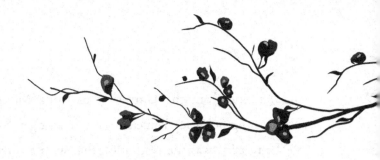

About the Author

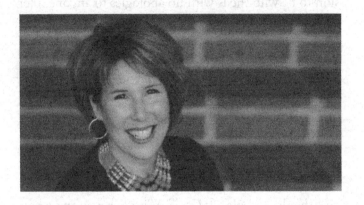

Severe life challenges brought **PAMELA HERZER, M.A.**, a deep understanding and connection to divine Love, which inspired her to launch her coaching practice, divine Love Alignment in 2007. Pamela's rich understanding of Love's ever-presence empowers her to help others face down and overcome debilitating challenges to experience healing and regeneration.

Pamela earned a master's degree in Spiritual Psychology with an emphasis in Consciousness, Health,

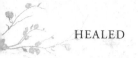

and Healing from the University of Santa Monica. The turning point for Pamela, to quote a slogan from the University, was the realization that we are "divine beings having a human experience." She learned how to take care of herself on the emotional, physical, mental, and spiritual levels. Finally, she gave herself permission to be who she is with no apologies to anyone. Her graduate work helped her to clear the past to make way for the future. She did this while staying in the present. Pamela was free to create a new life for herself with her hand in divine Love's.

When Pamela was diagnosed with cancer, pure gratitude for life that got her out of that pit of despair. In her words, "If I have ten more minutes to live, I will give thanks and glorify God." With her new awareness of the power of prayer to bring one into alignment with divine Love, she now commits her time to coaching and counseling others.

Pamela lives in Laguna Beach, California, with her husband, Todd. What brings her the most joy is being with family.

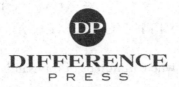

About Difference Press

Difference Press is the exclusive publishing arm of The Author Incubator, an educational company for entrepreneurs – including life coaches, healers, consultants, and community leaders – looking for a comprehensive solution to get their books written, published, and promoted. Its founder, Dr. Angela Lauria, has been bringing to life the literary ventures of hundreds of authors-in-transformation since 1994.

A boutique-style self-publishing service for clients of The Author Incubator, Difference Press boasts a fair and easy-to-understand profit structure, low-priced author copies, and author-friendly contract terms. Most importantly, all of our #incubatedauthors maintain ownership of their copyright at all times.

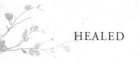

LET'S START A MOVEMENT
WITH YOUR MESSAGE

In a market where hundreds of thousands of books are published every year and are never heard from again, The Author Incubator is different. Not only do all Difference Press books reach Amazon bestseller status, but all of our authors are actively changing lives and making a difference.

Since launching in 2013, we've served over 500 authors who came to us with an idea for a book and were able to write it and get it self-published in less than 6 months. In addition, more than 100 of those books were picked up by traditional publishers and are now available in book stores. We do this by selecting the highest quality and highest potential applicants for our future programs.

Our program doesn't only teach you how to write a book – our team of coaches, developmental editors, copy editors, art directors, and marketing experts incubate you from having a book idea to being a published, bestselling author, ensuring that the book you create can actually make a difference in the world. Then we give you the training you need to use your book to make the difference in the world, or to create a business out of serving your readers.

ARE YOU READY TO MAKE A DIFFERENCE?

You've seen other people make a difference with a book. Now it's your turn. If you are ready to stop watching and start taking massive action, go to http://theauthorincubator.com/apply/.

"Yes, I'm ready!"

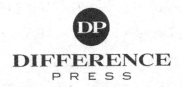

DIFFERENCE
P R E S S

Other Books by Difference Press

What Happened to My Happily Ever After?:
The Radical Approach to Revitalize Your Marriage
or Divorce with Love by Belinda Zylberman

Stop Hating Your Body: Healing Anorexia for Good
by Sarah Hauch

My Family Needs My Spiritual Leadership Now:
The Guide to Being Your Family's Spiritual Support
by Kristin Panek

Love: The Women's Guide to Not F*cking Settling
by Carlen Costa

Ultimate Intimacy: The Revolutionary Science of Female
Sexual Health by Carolyn DeLucia

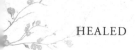

Promote Your Inner Cowgirl: The Horse Lover's Way to Work Less, Earn More, and Live Your Passion by Lynda Flowers

Winning Your Parents' Approval After Divorce: 7 Practices to Leave Your Marriage with Their Blessing by Cindy Gunraj

Feel Sexy Again: The Ultimate Guide to Reclaiming Your Sexual Confidence by Erica Lemke-Pembroke

I Ain't Thinking About You: The 8-Step Guide to Finally Letting Him Go Using the Breakup Funeral Method by Lenina Mortimer

It's Hard! Sexual Satisfaction Secrets to Beat Erectile Dysfunction by S. Sequoia Stafford

I Can Sit Again: Clinically Proven Treatment for Tailbone Pain by Jennifer Stebbing

Love Your Body: The Ultimate Guide to Stop Making Your Body a Battleground by Janet Farnsworth